BORN TO LIVE

GLADYS TAYLOR McGAREY, M.D. M.D. (H)

Foreword by Elisabeth Kubler-Ross, M.D.

INKWELL PRODUCTIONS®
Scottsdale, Arizona
www.inkwellproductions.com

First printing July 2008

ISBN: 978-0-9814648-4-X
Library of Congress Control Number: : 2008934643

Published by Inkwell Productions
10869 N. Scottsdale Road # 103-128
Scottsdale, AZ 85254-5280

Tel. 480-315-3781
E-mail: info@inkwellproductions.com
Website: www.inkwellproductions.com

Other works by Dr. Gladys McGarey,
The Physician Within You

Also her amazing biography written masterfully by Analea McGarey,
Born to Heal

Coming soon, Dr. McGarey's new book,
Living Medicine

Printed in the United States of America

Acknowledgments

To the hundreds of women who have written their stories for me and who have expressed a desire of sharing their stories with others. I have only been able to include a very small number of their stories in this book but the richness of the information shared with me permeates every page. And to my ex-husband, William McGarey, who made the first publication of this book a possibility.

Especially to Betsy, who will be a fourth generation woman physician, and has worked closely with me in the republication of this book.

To Doris Solbrig, who has spent countless hours of dedicated assistance in this revision.

To my grandson Daniel Wechsler who re-typed this whole manuscript.

And finally I also acknowledge the ongoing help of my publisher Nick Ligidakis who supported and encouraged me to republish this book.

The cover was designed by Eric Espamer and Jamie Davis, who gave us permission to photograph her 2 week old baby Estelle as, "the star."

Contents

Foreword

It is a great privilege and delight for me as well as an honor and a challenge to write a foreword to this book on birth, death, life, beginnings and endings. It is probably one of the first books of the New Age written by a physician with a life-long experience in beginnings and ending. She is herself a remarkable woman who has shown an incredible sensitivity, openness and awareness, which comes only through personal growth, endless observation and an open mind, a searching for the truth and a willingness to step out of the ordinary paths to find new questions and new answers.

I have known Gladys McGarey for thirty years. Since I have specialized in the ending of the physical existence and she has become an expert in the beginnings of this physical life, we formed an immediate affinity to each other and discovered that both of us, although in a different language perhaps, talked about the same experiences. Since birth is a transition from the spiritual existence to the physical world, so is death a step out of the physical world and a re-entry into the spiritual realm of which we are just beginning to know more and more.

This book begins with an explanation of our inability to have any recall whence we came and describes it in a form of an angel of forgetfulness, who gently touches us the moment we decide to begin life again.

And life naturally begins when the soul, the entity, enters the physical body to start a new existence in the physical world. We are here to grow, to learn, to have all the positive experiences that the physical world can offer. And when we have passed all the tests, we are allowed to graduate and return back to our original home.

We are endowed with all the assets for a total life experience and are able to fulfill those experiences in one lifetime, though very few people are able to do that. It is important to understand that human beings consist of a physical, emotional, spiritual and intellectual quadrant and that only if those four are in harmony and inter-balanced with each other that we can stay whole and healthy and fulfill our destiny.

Gladys gives beautiful examples of people's fears and anxieties, of their inner awareness, of expanded consciousness, of their intuitive knowledge of things to happen, and brings beautiful stories of special children whom we never give enough credit since often when the physical, intellectual quadrant is handicapped, the spiritual, intuitive quadrant becomes more the functioning, and many of these children rely on their own deep inner knowledge. They are indeed special children who touch many lives in their short existence and help parents and caretakers to grow far beyond anything they would have experienced had it not been for the short life span of these special children.

Born to Live makes a plea for home care, just as we have made a plea for allowing patients to die at home. And in reading through these pages I am once more reminded how terribly identical the moment of birth is to the moment of death, when you enter from a dark place, through a tunnel towards the light, expected and welcomed by the warm, caring hands of those who took care of us on both sides of this invisible barrier.

Gladys McGarey also has the courage to talk openly and frankly about her envolving concepts of abortion, and as a woman who was married for decades and has been studying, not only the Bible, but the Cayce material, she brings about some interesting and fascinating new concepts, which are important to study, to evaluate, and to form an opinion on. It is sad that most of our life is spent in criticizing, labeling, and judging other people's behavior and concepts by breeding more fear, guilt and shame rather than looking within ourselves and wondering why we have to point our fingers at others in order to deflect the attention from our own negativity.

Anyone who is willing to read Gladys' book with an open mind and a heart full of love, understanding and wisdom will be grateful for her courage and will learn a great deal, not only about beginning and ending, but about life itself.

Thank you, Gladys, for the warm and personal sharing, and for the courage you have to let more people know about the real meaning of unconditional love.

Elisabeth Kubler-Ross, M.D.

Preface

This book is a collection of real life stories about birth and life in the New Age. It is a string of precious beads in which the thread holding them together is woven of my own interpretive abilities and my philosophy.

As often as possible, I have quoted the stories as the individuals experiencing the events wrote them for me. Other stories are in my own words, as nearly as I could remember them as they were told to me. And the remainder of the tales told are from my own experience in the area of delivering babies into the world and taking care of people and their problems in the course of my practice in medicine. My interpretation of the meaning of all these life experiences is just that.

I hope these pages will speak for themselves, and perhaps my readers – as they move through these life-changing happenings – will find their own interpretations bringing new meaning and direction to their own lives.

The philosophy holding things together here for me is based on my own experience and heritage, and enriched by my study of the Bible and the information I found in fifty-five years of close association and work with the Edgar Cayce psychic readings. The Cayce material brought a richness and depth into my previous commitment to the Bible story.

The format of this book grew out of long conversations I've had with my younger daughter Helene. Now grown, she is my partner in the practice of medicine. Since she was a child, Helene has had her heart set on being a doctor, so we found an easy free communication growing with the years. As she left home for college,

Helene was not near at hand, and I had less opportunity to carry on these communications. Thus, I found that stories I wanted to tell, and thoughts I longed to share, moved into the shadows of the past often without a voice.

This book, then, may help to capture some of those fleeting moments in time and help to correct the situation with Helene, to give her some of the beauty I've found in other peoples' lives, and perhaps, to give her some base of understanding that has helped to make my practice of medicine a lifetime of joy and wonder. The book is not directed only to Helene, but to every daughter whose future looms ahead on the horizon as an exciting mysterious encounter with Life itself, an adventure worth pursuing. And it is dedicated to every individual in this world who sees in birth, life and death the mystery of the adventure of one's soul passing through time and space, leading towards a goal which we often perceive only in the dim light of the future.

I am no longer delivering babies and, much to her disappointment, neither is Helene. The medical practice has shifted enough that it is not possible for us to do so. However, it has not diminished my interest in the whole process of birth and birthing.

The material in this book remains as relevant today as it was in 1980 and, therefore, with some additions I choose to republish at this time.

Dedication

This book is dedicated to my parents who created the opportunity for me to be born in India and allowed me to grow up in a loving home filled with humor and deep faith in God and my fellow human being.

To my children who have taught me lessons from the moment they were conceived to the present day and who each one has become healers in their own right.

To my grandchildren who are the light of my life, especially to Betsy, a fourth generation woman physician who has worked closely with me for the republication of this book.

To Doris Solbrig who has spent countless hours of dedicated assistance in these revisions.

To my patients whose lives have deeply touched and influenced mine and whose stories I am sharing with the reader.

To the hundreds of women who have written their stories for me and who have expressed a desire in sharing their stories with others. I have only been able to include a very small number of their stories in this book but the richness of the information shared with me permeates every page.

To my ex-husband, William McGarey, who made the first publication of this book a possibility.

To Virginia Benderly who made the republishing of this book feasible and finally to Nick Ligidakis, my publisher, who has worked patiently with me through the last two revisions.

The Mystery of the Human Hand

The human hand has always been a fascination for me. However, when I was young my hands were an embarrassment. My sister's hands were beautiful with long slender fingers. My hands were big and square and every year when I was in school at Woodstock in the Himalayas, when winter came on, I had chilblains severe enough that my fingers were swollen and itchy and cracked and bleeding and my hands were ugly. When I left India and came to the United States to start college, they were still an embarrassment to me. Other girls were able to paint their fingernails and have beautiful dainty hands but mine were big and square. I would not put nail polish on them. In fact, in order not to call attention to them, I would frequently sit on my hands. This continued until I was well along in medical school and one day I saw a senior resident scrubbing up for surgery and as I watched her scrub, I said to myself, "Her hands are bigger that yours. Why are you ashamed of yours? They work. They're strong. Stop it," and I did. I stopped being ashamed of my hands and was grateful for the work I could do with them. It was the real epiphany. Later when I was doing deliveries and scrubbed up for delivery I always sang to myself the hymn, "Take my hands and let them be consecrated Lord to Thee." I did the same when I scrubbed for surgery. Soon my hands became an integral part of my practice in medicine.

Recently it became necessary to republish *Born To Live*. Since I never have been pleased with covers I used for earlier editions it was necessary to create a new cover. I wanted a picture on the cover to show two strong hands holding a newborn baby. I thought of several people with strong hands, who could pose for the picture, but then I became aware that maybe my hands should be the ones photographed. I also realized that when we did the cover for *Born To Heal* my hand is on the bottom, my granddaughter's hand is on top of that and my Hindustani sister's hand on top of that and my hand really does not show. I realized that the time has come for me to acknowledge my hands for what they are, glory in the fact that they not only work, but also have been blessed to welcome newborn babies. So this new cover shows my hands holding baby Estelle, a two-week-old beautiful little baby girl.

The lesson I have learned is that the parts of my body, which I was ashamed of, have become a thing of beauty because they have been dedicated to service and love.

CHAPTER ONE

The Angel of Forgetfulness

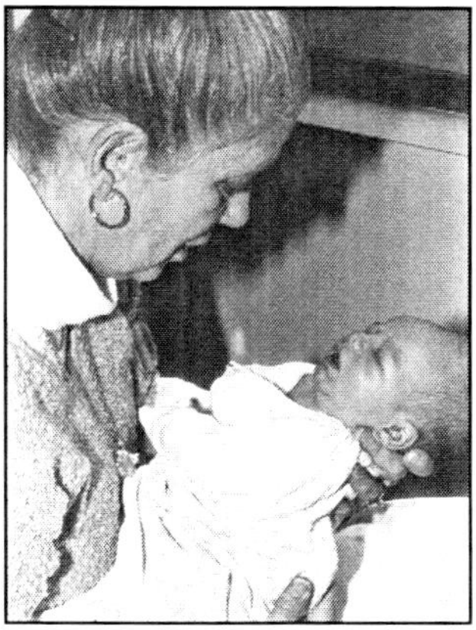

Birthing in the New Age creates several very fascinating questions. One finds its way out of ages past, when perhaps the earth was much younger, but children were still being born. The new life with its joys and its wonders excited the imagination of the mother and she would whisper in her inner mind, "Where does this wonderful miracle come from?"

In our travels, seeking for new adventures and relationships, Bill and I found ourselves in the study of Rabbi Herbert Weiner in South Orange, New Jersey, shortly after the Sabbath services had ended. We were meeting him for the first time, and we were interested in bringing the Rabbi out to Council Grove, Kansas, for a special interdisciplinary meeting of clinicians, researchers, scientists and authors. And, we were bandying ideas about.

The subject of rebirth came up, quite naturally, I am sure, for Bill and I thought in those terms most of the time in our effort to get this intricate life into some perspective. We knew, also, that Rabbi Weiner was an authority on the Kabbala, having researched and written books and articles on the subject.

"From our tradition," the rabbi began, "there is a fascinating story I'm sure would interest you. It is said that before a person is born, he carries a light on his head, which enables him to see from one end of creation to another. Perhaps that means he is given a full picture, a preview of all the things that are going to happen to him in life ahead. All the good things and the bad, all the difficulties and the accomplishments, the joys and sorrows, the highs and the lows, those individuals whom he will spend time with – the whole story.

Then he is told that he must choose, for choice is always one of man's sacred gifts from the Creator, and the final choice is his. If, then, the answer is 'Yes' – the Angel of Forgetfulness touches him on the center of his upper lip and he forgets everything he saw, and he is born."

The Rabbi smiled, and we all felt quite comfortable, for isn't it nice to have ideas about how we do indeed come into the world, and have them backed up by a tradition? His tradition is a bit different from mine, and neither of them find any scientific basis to back them up. But, fortunately for both of us, and for the scientific discipline (and its adherents), the Creator has established laws which are as yet not discovered, not recognized, and which are undoubtedly above anything the world of science might prove or disprove.

It seemed to me as we continued our visit with this warm, gentle man that the assumptions he made might be carried a bit farther. If, indeed, there is an Angel of Forgetfulness and each of us gets the opportunity to choose where we will be born, then we must also ask the question, "How did we get there in the first place, so that we might choose?"

If we agreed that we were created in the spiritual realms as a spiritual being, then, there are several possibilities. Either we were about to enter the earth plane for the first time through being born, or we were entering back into the realm we know as "life" here on earth for the second or the third time (or more), having died to this life prior to spending an interim in the spiritual realm. That's what is commonly called reincarnation.

We left the Rabbi's study, after beginning a friendship that has intensified through the years, but we continued our thinking and our discussion about this strange thing that involves the life process, this event known as "rebirth."

To be "reborn" has special spiritual significance here in the Western World in the minds and the lives of those who hold the traditional Christian concept from the Bible. In this context, there is a presupposition that a soul seeks to understand and to grow spiritually. This rebirth experience is an elevating, enlightening event, sometimes occurring in the midst of a full and satisfied life. It is meaningful to the participant and changes the manner in which he lives his life as the years go by.

To the Eastern mind, however, and increasingly common now to millions of people in our part of the world, is the idea that to be reborn is another physical birth. Rebirth, in this sense of the word, is that occasion when a person or an entity – a soul, the spiritual essence, the ongoing individual reality – makes that transition from the spiritual realm to be born into a new physical body into the material life once again.

This idea of what we call reincarnation seems to tell us that the spiritual realm (the fourth dimension, the inter-between, the "place" where we go when we die, the living experience that we take part in before we are born) is our true home, the origin of our being, the domain of what we call God, the Creator.

When a child is born, it is such a natural thing for one to wonder and dream about the origin of that little bundle of human flesh, two cells united and became one; then divided, shaped, communicated and started functioning to become a living human individual with potential far greater than our minds can even grasp.

This concept of repeated earth lives implies several things. Not only is there a continuity of the being that we call "I," but also there is a purpose, a need for learning, a possibility of experiencing and growing spiritually. If the spiritual realms are truly our origin, then aren't they also our destiny (in some way we find hard to conceive of)? Is it not possible too, that our goal is a oneness with that which we call the Creator, though we must also maintain our own individuality, remember all things, and set to rest the conflicts, wars, and self-desires that separate us from that destiny.

For some fifty-five years, I have been studying, researching and using concepts found in the Edgar Cayce psychic data, as I both practiced medicine and shared things with my six children.

Edgar Cayce was a humble man who died in 1945 in Virginia Beach, Virginia. He is perhaps the most well known and certainly the most well documented physic of our time. He had the astonishing ability to be able to move into an altered state of consciousness and contact the unconscious mind of the person for whom he was giving a "reading." There are 14,000 of these readings, which have been studied in detail and are housed in Virginia Beach, Virginia. For most of his lifetime, people would write to him giving their name and address and ask for help for all manner of problems, physical, mental, emotional, and spiritual. He then, from this state of altered consciousness, gave them readings explaining why the condition existed and what they could do about it. Some 9,000 of the readings were what have been termed physical readings which meant that they dealt with physical problems. These dealt with aspects of disease and therapeutic modalities which were sometimes unusual and other times very conventional for the time. The depth and breadth of this work has been an ongoing source of information and inspiration to me.

When the idea of reincarnation became part of my thinking I already had four children. Helene and David, however, came into our home after I had learned something about how to prepare for pregnancy, and what life may be about after all. Helene is nearly three years older than David. Both of them talked about possible past lives as easily as they discussed classmates in school. But, it seemed that emotions always played their part, and Helene picked on David from the time he was little. They became the best of friends in the later teen years, but those early years were sometimes stressful.

It was during one of these episodes that the two of them really got into a fuss. David usually handled Helene's "pickiness" with equanimity, but not this time. As Bill and I pulled them apart, he took Helene to one side, and I marched David into the other room.

"Helene, you know you have to learn to live with David," Bill sternly lectured her. "If you don't make peace with him this time, you may come back having to live with him as his wife. You know you chose to be born into this family!"

"Yes," she replied quick as a flash, "but that was before I knew David was coming."

It's been a learning experience for both of them, and happily they have gained a great deal from their relationship. If, indeed, something from a past life had to be learned, then set to rest, they have accomplished it.

Our study of the Cayce readings brought this selection to our attention. It seems to speak to this learning experience of our two younger children:

> Know that each sojourn of indwelling may be compared to that as ye have in your mental experience as a lesson, as a schooling for the purposes for which each soul-entity enters an earth experience; and why an entity under such environments come into that experience. 1158-5

Another way to put things is to see Helene and David being born into the same family in order to gain the opportunity to choose the right manner when things of a "karmic" or past-life nature come about. Karma, the law of cause and effect (what you sow you will also reap) brings into one's life a test, a possibility of overcoming, for completing a cycle that the soul has set into motion.

Bill and I continued our research on how children come into this world and why it is that most of us don't remember anything prior to our being born, and I also puzzled a bit over my own experience. I don't really recall my birth experience – maybe the Angel of Forgetfulness was highly efficient with me – and it wasn't until my forty-ninth year that a memory pattern flooded into my conscious mind. It really had an impact, and it happened while we were on a round-the-world tour with a large group of people, visiting India, where we interviewed a number of people who had remembered parts of their past lives.

But let me go back a bit. I do remember, and my family keeps reminding me, that when I was two years old, I announced that I was going to be a doctor. The fact that my mother and father were both physicians may have had something to do with it, but that certainly was not all. I never desired to do anything else. All my energies seemed directed towards this goal.

When I was in college, my mother used to write to me and suggest that I take some teacher training courses. My grades weren't at the top of the class and it didn't seem likely that I would ever get accepted into the medical school. Yet, my decision never wavered – it was like a burning need, almost as though I had some vow to fulfill. I never did take those teacher training courses, and I did get into medical school.

My interests have always been in obstetrics. I loved general practice, but bringing babies into the world had been most important and an integral portion of my whole experience in medicine. After fifty years in the field, I still became very much involved in the lives of my O.B. patients as well as in the deliveries themselves. I worked through the difficult parts with each patient, and even seemed to draw the abnormal presentations, the complications, and the difficulties to me as though it were part of what I would expect. Bill used to wonder, over and over again, when he was also delivering babies, why he would get the normal O.B.s and I would always have the difficult problems. It was uncanny, the way it happened.

My parents were both medical missionaries in India, spending over fifty years in the field, and birthing most of us (my three brothers, my sister and myself) there in India.

In 1920 mother and dad figured it was about time for me to come into this world. So they left their missionary compound in Roorkee, United Province, and drove towards the Presbyterian Hospital in Fatehgarh, which is twenty-four miles northwest of Agra – not far from the location of the Taj Mahal.

They wanted to see the Taj and thought it would be nice to let the other children see this marvel of construction, so they planned their trip with this in mind. Roads being what they were in those days, and our model "T" Ford being what it was, the trip was not easy.

Just as they drove up and got out of the car, Mother felt a bit strange. Then, as they came into full view of the magnificent Taj Mahal, mother had her first labor pain. Since it was her fourth pregnancy, they both knew that they had to move quickly and get to the hospital. The roads were rough and rutted but they made it in time for me to arrive in the hospital, and not on the road.

Dr. Woodward, a wonderful old lady physician, was the officiating member of the party as I made my grand entrance, and all went well.

Just after I was born, however, Dr. Woodward had to leave for Calcutta since she needed to have some laboratory tests done on herself, and they were not available there in the Presbyterian Hospital in Fatehgarh. After she left, the cook in the room next to where mother was bedded dropped a teakettle accidentally on the floor. The noise was so loud and so startled my mother that she jumped out of bed to see what had happened.

Her precipitous ambulation was not good – she started hemorrhaging and there was much difficulty in getting the flooding stopped. After much delay, Dr. Woodward finally returned, surgically packed the uterus, and the bleeding stopped. Mother made a slow and otherwise uneventful recovery.

Because of her blood loss and the weakness that followed (there were no blood transfusions available for her at that time) mother was unable to feed me at breast. I was the only one of her five children whom she was not able to nurse, and I think it is interesting that I have never liked milk to this day. Also, I rarely drink it – then only if it is disguised.

Dad scouted around through the small town of Fatehgarh looking for what might be appropriate to use as a nursing bottle, until he found a little pewter toy teapot (see photo at the end of chapter) much like the teapots which were used for many, many centuries in India. He tied the rubber end of a medicine dropper to the spout, poked a hole in the end of a rubber device, and presented me with my first baby bottle. I drank buffalo's milk as an infant, much as children of India have done for hundreds of years if their mother's milk was not available to them. One of my prized possessions to this day is that little baby bottle, just as good now as it was then.

I have thought often about what has been called the "Akashic Records." This seems to be the storehouse of all the things that have happened in those many lifetimes each individual experiences. It can be drawn upon, by those who are qualified to do so. How one gets that privilege is not clear.

The Akasha has been likened to a tapestry, which we weave through the thoughts and acts we bring into being through our relations with other people, through what we do about what we know is right to do, and through those things that fail to measure up to the standards we have set for ourselves. The tapestry is like a pattern that we have created, and if we could see it, we could perhaps interpret at least part of what we see. But, like a real tapestry in the earth plane, it is made up of the somber tones of sorrow as well as the golden ones of joy and love. The intricate pattern takes an expert to interpret fully.

Perhaps, in light of my own Akasha, it was not just a coincidence that mother went into labor with me when she saw the Taj. It was probably an important event in my total life picture and in her own weaving of the tapestry. Not only did the Taj herald my birth, in a sense, but also, I was the only child in my family with whom mom had any complications – that being a severe postpartum hemorrhage. I had to drink buffalo milk out of an ancient teapot that brought the distant past into the present for me. In other words, from what I've learned, my birth may have been saying things to me symbolically, that I did not really understand until forty-nine years later.

Then, back again on the tour, we were in a bus, in Agra, and the bus driver was telling the story of how and why the Taj was built. Shah Jahan had built the Taj Mahal as a memorial for his beautiful wife, Mum Taz Mahal, who had gone out to the battlefield with the Shah. She was pregnant with her fourteenth child, and delivered in a tent while out near the battlefield. After the birth of the child, she hemorrhaged, the midwife was unable to stop the bleeding, and she died.

As I listened to the story, I felt as though someone had stuck a hot poker up my back. I was startled by my own reaction then, never having felt anything like that before.

After the bus stopped, we disembarked and walked to the great gates. There in front of us, in all its wonderful magnificence and glory, stood the Taj Mahal. I started to cry. Bill approached me and asked what was wrong. I told him not to bother me, continued to cry and walked off by myself. I didn't know why I was crying, but I couldn't seem to stop. We toured through the tomb – for it was a tomb for Mum Taz Mahal – and my tears continued.

It was mid-afternoon by the time we returned to the hotel. I was tired and I decided that I really wanted to take a nap. I fell into a deep sleep and I do not remember what I dreamed, but I awakened saying to myself, "Why do you feel so badly – you helped her through thirteen. She died with the fourteenth." It was then that I realized that I had been the midwife who delivered babies for Mum Taz Mahal. She died from postpartum hemorrhage. The next day, traveling around Agra, we arrived on the spot where Shah Jahan held court and sentenced those who had broken the law. Again the tears came – just like the experience at the Taj. Then I thought, "What sort of fate would lie in wait for the midwife who would allow Mum Taz Mahal to die? What was my fate in that lifetime?" Those who were sentenced to die lost their heads.

If the story has reality as part of its impact, it is then understandable that the circumstances and events of my birth were more than just coincidence. Could it be, for reasons established in that lifetime, that I would be born in this lifetime into a family where my parents were not only both physicians, but also missionaries to India? That I would be born just twenty-four miles from the Taj Mahal? It seems also reasonable and logical, given that my story is real, that my mother would almost die from hemorrhage and become unable to breast feed me, thus making it necessary for me to feed from a makeshift teapot like those used in India hundreds of years ago.

Events of the distant past can be instructive and helpful, but are often disturbing and sometimes downright painful. It is undoubtedly a blessing for most of us that the Angel of Forgetfulness lets us forget not only what is coming, but also what has already happened, when we are born.

Therefore, as we examine this newborn child of the New Age, we may not know from where he had his origins in experience. We can know, however, that much is hidden behind those searching eyes that reach up to make contact with the light. The potential of this little one is well beyond our wildest imaginings.

Pewter toy teapot

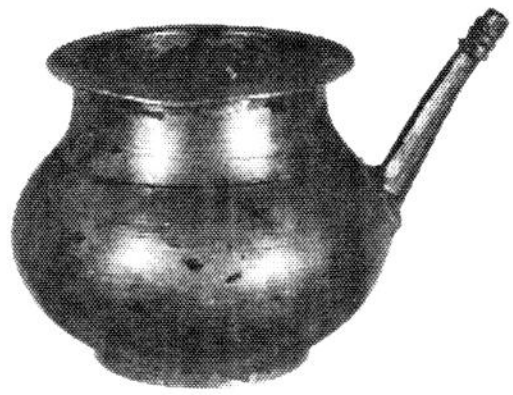

CHAPTER TWO

Old Wine in New Wineskins

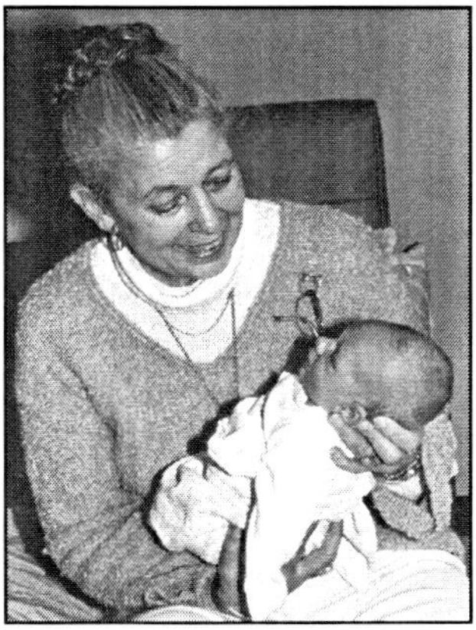

My experience with the Taj Mahal, with all its implications, helped me to understand that birth and death are really different aspects of the same process. I died in that incarnation, taking with me the memories and experiences of those times and those events that became such an important part of me then, and I was born into the spiritual spheres. What goes on there is another subject, and I don't claim to be at all informed about that. But, after a lapse of what we call time in that dimension, I was born back into the earth plane, and died to the spiritual. My memories persisted, although they were now deep in my unconscious mind, waiting to be interpreted from the tapestry of the Akasha that we all weave.

In the Bible, Jesus tells the parable about the wineskin. He admonishes us not to put new wine in old wineskins. The way I interpret that is perhaps that we should not try to fit new concepts to old ways of thinking. It won't work.

But the idea of old wine being placed in new wineskins fits admirably with the idea of reincarnation and the continuity of life. For we are indeed old wine, having brought the flavor with us from many past incarnations. Each lifetime, however, presents us with a new body, a new environment to work with – a new wineskin.

One day while shopping I saw a mother and daughter walk by, adding foods to their cart as they moved through the aisles of the supermarket. I caught my breath, for the two of them looked, for all the world, like Egyptian princesses. The sharp, yet well contoured, clear faces, the black hair, cut Egyptian style, the manner in which they walked – all this spoke so clearly of Egypt, that I really marveled at that resemblance. They moved on, and I forgot the instance, for a few months.

In my office, several months later, I walked into one of my examining rooms to see my next patient, and again I caught my breath. There was the mother Egyptian princess with her daughter-princess waiting to be seen. The problem? The girl, perhaps five years old, was having nightmares. They had been persisting for several weeks, and nothing the mother could do would relieve the situation. The dreams were all the same, and the child would awaken screaming; she was being attacked by swarms of flies and frogs. Over and over again the nightmare would recur, and over and over again the flies and frogs would come back.

I questioned the mother. She had never read her daughter the story of the plagues that were visited on the Egyptians when Moses was trying to get the Pharaoh to let the children of Israel go. She had never told her anything about the plagues, was not really very familiar with the story herself.

Was this past-life memory of an event which really happened to the child? Was it part of the flavor of the wine that had been poured into this new wineskin? We certainly can't prove it one way or another, but one thing was certain, there was at least a solution to the problem.

The mother was instructed to talk to the child gently and reassuringly as she went to sleep each night and at that time particularly when she entered the first stages of deep sleep. During that period, the mother assured the girl that she was loved and that she would be all right. After about two weeks, the nightmares never recurred.

Perhaps the little Egyptian princess experienced a lifetime in Egypt and died in the plagues, but if so, the memory of the event is laid to rest with love and caring and the gentle attention given by her mother.

From the Cayce material, a great deal can be gained dealing with lives of trauma and new births, which allow the trauma to be set at rest. The mechanism involves both birth and death, the two sides of the coin when one considers life and what it means. In one of the readings, Cayce said it like this:

> "The passing in, the passing out, is as but the summer, the fall, the spring: the birth into the interim, the birth into the material." 281-16

Birth into the material is certainly more than someone having a baby and someone officiating at the delivery of the newcomer. It does involve physical aspects of movement in consciousness.

From the search currently being done by those studying biofeedback and the changes that come in the electroencephalogram with the varying degrees of control one has over his own unconscious functions, we can understand that we are continually moving from one state of consciousness to another.

In our own life experience, while we sleep, for instance, we recognize that we are in one state of awareness that we call the sleep and dream state. That is one state of consciousness. The waking state is another, much different, level of consciousness.

Other states are recognizable, like the way we listen to someone's rather dull conversation, our eyes a bit glazed and our minds occupied with not only the person's voice and subject material, but also the boat trip we took last month, or the show on TV that was so good, or how our kids are getting along back East. The kitchen sink state of consciousness might be more easily recognizable – the kaleidoscope of mental images and imaginings that move through one's mind as one washes a mountain of dishes.

Birth is much like that. It is a change of consciousness, a change from a spiritual into a physical environment. Much like moving from one room into another, physically. One experiences different things; one sees a completely new set of circumstances, one finds within a wholly changed set of feelings and awareness. Being eternal beings, we move from the world of creation into the created world.

I like to think of birth as a change comparable to that which today's airport experience can provide. In 1955, our four children and I joined Bill out in Phoenix, moving from Wellsville, Ohio. We flew from the Pittsburgh airport at 8:00 a.m., leaving behind our friends and relatives who were there to see us off. Later on that afternoon, at about 4:30 p.m., we arrived in Phoenix and a welcoming party headed up by my husband greeted us. What a contrast – lush summer greenness of the Ohio and Pennsylvania hills, which we left behind, and the hot, sunny, sandy desert land of Arizona. Birth is like that, isn't?

Since those days, having lived in Phoenix, I don't often think back to Wellsville, unless something specifically reminds me to do so. But, I can and do reminisce, recalling how it was on a Sunday morning, to walk down the concrete steps from that front porch of our house on Aten Avenue, around the corner past the Roberts' house, and on another half block to the church. Most of the time, however, I am involved with the events as they occur here in our present living environment. Our seven years in Wellsville could just as well have been a dream.

How does that fit with the birth of a baby? Or the death of a baby? This is much like the analogy of the airports. People gather around the one who is dying to wish that soul bon voyage with love. We spend time in the realm of the spirit, and then when that soul arrives back on the earth plane (again like the airplane voyage) there is a welcoming party of loved ones to greet him, and say, "Here's a whole new life for you." It's only in dreams, meditations, visions or other altered states of awareness that one recalls where he has come from.

I found the airport story to be helpful in working with the women who came to me for obstetrical care. I had told them this story, and then quite often, when labor came and the patient was ready to deliver, we put her legs in the stirrups, and I would say, "O.K. let's fasten our seat belts, because we're coming in for a landing."

If birth is like coming in for a landing, then death is like taking off for parts at least partially unknown – the other side of the coin.

Esther met me for lunch one day, and in the course of our conversation, she told me the story of the grocery store door. Her brother-in-law owned a grocery store in the heart of a small town in Illinois. Bob had lived there all his life, and his store was an integral part of the small town's activities. He and his wife were dearly loved by the neighbors and by their customers.

One day, Esther's sister-in-law called to report that Bob had suffered a stroke. He was placed in the hospital, and tests were performed to clarify his condition, because he was not responding well. Customers brought Bob's wife their condolences, and knew that Bob had been hospitalized with a stroke.

However, as time wore on, the tests revealed that it was not a stroke at all, but a brain tumor, and he was not really expected to live much longer. Shocked, the family chose not to tell their customers this new bit of information. For some reason or another, they felt that they didn't want to burden the customers with the news.

One morning, the wife was opening the store and, as she unlocked the door, it fell right off its hinges. News of this spread though the town and people began streaming into the store, offering their condolences. This incident of the door falling off its hinges symbolized to these people that Bob was going to die – and, within a week, Bob died.

Symbols, like distant memories, seem to speak to the unconscious mind of man, and become meaningful when the need is there. Bob was leaving and many of his friends became aware that the departure flight was not far off and they gathered to wish him well and see him off.

It seems to me that, in order to appreciate birth to its fullest extent, and the reality that exists on both sides of a child's entry into the world, one must also appreciate the death event.

The Biblical student will recall that Paul longed for that state that comes after death – many times this was his wish. The story of Jesus is one where life in death is as clear and distinct as life in what we call life. While he certainly did not relish the kind of death he was facing, Jesus was able (if we can accept the Cayce story of his crucifixion) to joke on his way to the cross.

Such an event is not wholly out of context with reality, as we know it. I remember how my mother died at eighty-nine years of age. She had spent nearly all her life in India as a medical missionary, and now she was in our home, ill and suffering from polycythemia vera, a severe blood disorder where there are too many red blood cells, a strange follow-up since she had almost hemorrhaged to death at my birth. The outlook was not good. She was nearly ninety years old and had said over and over again that she was tired. I think she was trying to tell us that she wanted to go.

Then, on the Thursday before Easter, she fell, walking with the aid of her cane, coming into her room from the outdoors, where she was enjoying the petunias that were in bloom. She fractured her knee, ribs and pelvis, was hospitalized and we obtained x-rays of her bony injuries. As we moved her onto the hard surface of the x-ray table, it obviously hurt her a great deal. She flinched with pain, knowing, I am sure, that she would not recover from this injury. She looked up and saw on my father's face and in mine the pain we were feeling with her, and wishing to ease it a little for us, her comment was, with a wry smile, "The old gray mare, she just ain't what she used to be!" She died on Good Friday.

My experience with the death process did not end there. Two years after mother died, Dad remarried. His new wife was a longtime friend who had been widowed several years before that. "Mother Daniels" was also in her eighties, and they had a wonderful two-and-a-half years together. Dad became ill, however, while they were back East, and he expressed the wish to be out in Phoenix with us. We met him at the plane, and Bill helped him off. He was so ill we thought we might need a stretcher. Being a very strong Scotch-Irish Presbyterian, however, and filled with a lot of that Presbyterian zeal, he pulled himself erect, walked off the plane and down the steps with just a bit of help. He was able, however, to stay at home only overnight before we had to put him in the hospital.

Two weeks later, he had not improved. Mother Daniels suddenly was impressed to cancel an appointment and said, "I have to get to the hospital. We've got to go there now!" My sister-in-law drove her down to the hospital, and when they saw Dad, they knew that he was about ready to make the transition. They released the night nurse so she could go to breakfast.

After a time, they realized Dad was sleeping. Mother Daniels began to sing quietly "When the Roll is Called Up Yonder, I'll be There," one of Dad's favorite hymns. His lips moved with hers as she sang. Then she moved to "God Be With You Till We Meet Again," and his lips continued to move with hers for a while – then they stopped. He had made the transition.

When I went to the hospital to pick up Mother Daniels and Irma (my sister-in-law), Mother Daniels said to me, through her tears, "Don't you know there is a jubilation on the other side?"

This is what the death process should be like. We should really be jubilant, not just sad because of our loss and because of the fact that we missed him tremendously, but happy because we knew that my own mother was waiting for him on the other side.

I was further confronted by another bit from the Cayce readings:

> "... That which we see manifested in the material plane is but a shadow of that in the spiritual plane." (5749-3)

What we call a "presence" here – not seeing it or feeling it, physically – may be the greater reality. Something to think about when we consider how a child is born, and what kind of "presence" we are welcoming to the earth plane.

Elisabeth Kubler-Ross has made the greatest impact on the thinking of the Western World about death with her research on people who have died and come back. They report being aware, feeling wonderful and moving towards a great, beautiful, beneficent light. They never reach the light, for they are brought back to the earth life, nearly all of them with the feeling that they still have something important to do.

Dr. Kubler-Ross tells the story in one of her lectures of how she remembers the feeling she had in utero, the feeling of being squashed – as if someone were sitting on her, and of being hardly able to move. This is not a death story, for Elizabeth was the first of triplets, and I would suppose the other two were perched on her shoulders most of the time, waiting to be born.

Her memory also relates how much she appreciated the love and tenderness, the warmth of the physician's caring hands, as she and her sisters were ushered into the world. I would think, if my father were aware, as he was delivered into that state of awareness in the spiritual realm, he appreciated the warm and caring attention of the welcoming party who had gathered on that side to aid in his transition as well as the love of those of us in this realm who "saw him off."

Extended states of consciousness are apparent for our observation in literally thousands of individuals today. We must expect them in the infants that are born into this world, as well as in adult individuals who come into awareness that they are more than they seem. It is not many who can remember their stay in utero. Not too many have the experience of dying and returning. Only some are able to recall past lives, and the number is not great of those who can psychically perceive others' illnesses or prior incarnations. Yet, adding all these individuals together, the number challenges the imaginations of those who manifest such abilities in the world today.

There are many levels of consciousness available to us, which we do not, most of the time, even recognize. We influence each other in so many ways, even as an infant or as a child, and these ways have to be called at the present time "psychic," although the capabilities we deal with at those times are more likely to be normal qualities of the New Age person. After I published this book for the first time, a lady from Australia wrote the following story to me:

> We lived in a small N.S.W. Country town till I was three months pregnant with my fourth baby; then we moved about nine hundred miles away. We had no photos of the N.S.W. house; only one of the elder children standing in the front veranda. Our other three children were five, three and one when we left N.S.W. We never went back to the town again.
>
> When my youngest daughter was about eleven years of age, we had moved again and were back in N.S.W. – on north coast – Coff Harbor. She started talking about the time the tank's stand collapsed and the laundry was full of water; about the design of the house in Robertson (the little country town, N.S.W.) – which incidentally she drew – exactly even to the small step down from the lounge to the little hall to the bathroom. She described in detail – what was in each room, where the boys slept – about the huge gray stone in the back yard (it was a large 5ft x 2ft 6in stump of a tree) – about the large pine trees in the back lane. The elder of our boys – who was five years old when we left there – and would be the only one with any recallable memory of the area – argued

about the design but my younger daughter was correct. Even my husband had forgotten about the tank stand collapsing but I hadn't. Now all this to me means she must have been around – in spirit – prior to birth.

I can tell you, the day of the discussion in Coffs made my hair stand on end – but since then, I fully accept what she has told us and believe it possible.

One of God's "special people" brought this extended consciousness forcibly to my mind. The story came from a nurse who wrote of this incident for me:

A sixteen-year-old Down's syndrome child was operated on for a "belly button" sterilization procedure. After the operation she kept saying she was going to the "recovery room." We, as "adults," kept reassuring her that she did not have to go back to the recovery room, but she kept on saying that was where she was going.

Finally, we did listen to her, hear what she was saying, and asked her, "Why? Why are you going to the recovery room?" Her reply: "I'm going to tell the people there that they are not going to die, that they are going to get well."

The head nurse at the hospital where she had her surgery is a personal friend and began to check this statement of Berta's. There were several patients who did actually "dream" of a young girl coming to talk to them reassuring them that they were going to get well – some even thinking Roberta was an Oriental child – she has tip tilt dark brown eyes and dark brown hair.

This went on for over two years. After it stopped, I asked her if she still went to the recovery room, she said, "No, I'm not needed there anymore." She did not volunteer what she is doing or where she is doing whatever it is that she is doing.

Children of the New Age may not all be what we ordinarily call "gifted," but they may indeed be more gifted than we realize, and we may have an opportunity to work with unusual children who have abilities to influence the world in ways that we will see only if we really look.

I had another nurse tell me to following story:

> I was night supervisor of Garden Hospital, a nursing home in San Francisco, several years ago. Among my older patients was a lady about ninety years old. She was very frail and could have died at any time, at least it seemed that way to me. Her son's visits were few and far between. One night around 11:30 p.m., as I made my rounds, she said, "I wish I could die, but I need to say goodbye to someone. My son has not been here for so long and I am tired. Would you kiss me goodbye?" I didn't really know how to handle this, so I reassured her and told her she would probably feel better in the morning.
>
> However, two more nights, the same question. On the third night, I thought, maybe she would rest better if I complied with her request – so I wiped the perspiration from her forehead and kissed her. She said goodbye to me and kissed my hand. In a few moments she died.
>
> I have never been sure whether saying goodbye had anything to do with her death, but at times I have felt very guilty.

I think the nurse did a wonderful thing with her goodbye kiss. If death is that kind of an experience, if we can meet death without being medicated into confusion, so we are still conscious and aware, then we can face it head on, and not be afraid. Death is a reality – one that we will all face in order to leave this dimension for another. Obviously, if the foregoing information is valid at all, death is something we experience every time we make the transition from one state to another, and birth is on the other end of the transition.

How much does the unborn infant influence the birth time and place? This question has occurred to me so often, and I gained an insight into the possibilities as I worked with an expectant mother who had come to Phoenix from the Northwest, as her husband sought employment here. They had made the move before the child was even conceived. Thus, if the unborn individual really did exert an influence, it was a major factor in his life pattern, and the influence came all from the other side. But, these things did come about.

The story really made its impact on me during the last six weeks of pregnancy. Every time the mother would come into the office, the baby was in a breech position. I would rotate the baby to a vertex (head) presentation, and send the mother out, a normal pregnancy waiting to be delivered. Each time, she would come back with the breech presenting once more. Gradually, I even taught her to rotate the baby herself, since it was the easiest rotation I had ever done.

This continued until she went into labor. By then, she was able to tell which position the baby was in, so when she called me at the start of her labor, I asked, "What position is the baby in now?" Her response came, "He is breech."

"Okay," I said, "we'll see what we can do."

When I arrived to the hospital, there was no problem in rotating him once more. He delivered in vertex position, and everything was fine. I didn't think anything more about it afterwards, but instead tucked the incident away as an interesting medical phenomenon.

When the mother brought the baby in after a month for his check up, she told me this story. "I don't know why," she said, "but this child has been the most frightened child I've ever seen. He just screams. Every so often he looks terrified and starts to scream. I haven't been able to do anything to quiet him down."

I counseled the mother and scheduled her to be seen in a week once more. When she came in, she told me that she finally simply put the baby down on the bed, in utter desperation, and said to him, "Look – I don't know what to do with you. I've tried everything I know, and it hasn't worked. You obviously are frightened and there's something wrong with you. What it is? How can I help?" No words came from the infant and I am sure she did not expect them.

But that night she had a dream. In the dream, she was watching a battle between a large group of white men on horseback and a band of Indians. The scene was the Superstition Mountains, near Phoenix, and the fight was going on perilously near a cliff. One of the Indians suddenly lost his balance near the edge and fell precipitously, end over end, down hundreds of feet and met his death in the canyon below. The mother, the dreamer, was standing in the dream near where the man's body landed. She walked over toward where she knew the man had died. As she approached him, he got up, grew smaller and smaller, and she recognized him as her newborn child.

Then, as she awakened and realized what she had dreamed, it all began to make sense – all the things that had led up to and during the pregnancy. First, she and her husband moved here to Phoenix for reasons they did not understand. Then she became pregnant after they arrived. Throughout the entire pregnancy, her husband had never been able to locate a job.

At this point, now, well after the baby's birth, they were ready to move back to Oregon because he still could not find a job. As she and I began to talk about the whole incident, we pieced together the bits of the puzzle. The prime actor in the whole show was the infant. Was he in his last lifetime an Indian who fell head over heels down a precipice to his death? Did he influence his would-be parents to come from the far Northwest down to the place of his accident, his terror? If so, then the repeated turning from vertex to breech, over and over again, was a repetition of his falling from the cliff, head over heels.

Even after that, he was still terrified, and when his mother understood what had happened, she talked to him as he was falling in asleep. "If that is what happened, then it happened. It's done, it's over with, and you don't need to go through that experience again. You've been born into a new life, and you don't need fear and terror any more. We love you and we will help all we can to get rid of all those emotions that are so troublesome."

After she talked to him like that, he never had any more trouble. He was no longer a frightened, screaming baby. He was happy and peaceful.

Arizona history tells about a group of blue uniformed men who climbed up a secret path to the top of Big Picacho, which is now located on U.S. Route 60-70, just before reaching Superior, Arizona. They were soldiers from a company "B" of Arizona Volunteers and they had cornered seventy-five Apaches on Big Picacho Cliff. Shots were fired. There were war whoops, and finally Indians jumped off the cliff and fell to the rocks below. Legend has it that fifty Indians were killed in the first volley and there were maybe twenty-five or so who jumped off the cliff rather than be taken prisoners.

For one month after this happened the Indian squaws gathered around the area to mourn, and legend has it that their tears, which flowed so profusely, were imbedded in the rock by the Great Spirit and these tears are still there. They are called Apache tears and are black rocks, black obsidian, which can be polished to a rare beauty and are used as jewelry, not only by the Indians but by many people living out in the West.

In 1969, I was part of a tour visiting various physic persons around the world. One of the most fascinating events of the trip was our visit with a Hindu accountant who is blonde, blue-eyed, and deals with his children in all the strictness and regimentation that is typical of the Germanic peoples. His parents, however, are Hindu and they had never seen any Europeans. They grew up isolated from most of the world in their little village in India, and their heritage was one hundred percent East Indian.

When the accountant was a very young child he told his sister stories about his immediate past life experience. The sister recorded the information and his story unfolded to us as we visited with these people.

The boy recalled in the life before this being a World War I German officer. He did not want to be fighting a war. He hated killing and destruction, and though he tried to avoid being part of it, he had no choice, finding himself in the midst of the fighting.

He vowed if he ever got out of this, he would live in a place where there was peace, not war. This became almost an obsession with him. He was killed when a bullet passed through his neck.

When he returned to earth he was born in the early 1920s in India, truly a place of peace, not war, a place where Gandhi taught the gospel of nonresistance and peace. But he was ostracized as a child because of his light hair and strange appearance – strange to the dark Indian skin and hair of the other boys. It was so difficult for him that he finally dyed his hair so he would not look so out of place. He grew up peacefully, however, and became a government accountant.

But the most amazing part of the story is not the fact that he looked like a German, or that he recalled the information about his most recent life. It was not the blond hair, blue eyes, the regimentation that was part of his life, nor even the fact that he was considered European, not Indian, when he visited in foreign lands as part of his travels for the Indian government.

The most amazing part of this story just has to be the scar on his neck. He was born with the scar there – I examined it myself and took pictures of it. The scar is an indented one, exactly the kind one would suspect would be caused by a bullet wound. This is where the little boy said he had been shot as a German soldier, and the scar marks the manner in which he died.

The concept that consciousness, memory, even in the cells of the body, persists into the next lifetime add considerably to our understanding of the human being, the nature of consciousness and the nature of memory, its creation and its location.

It is reasonable, I think, if we put all these stories together with other information that we have at hand, to believe that we are in reality dealing with a ready-formed individual personality when we usher a baby into this world. We never know whether the baby is coming from a past life as a composer, a farmer, a genius of sorts, or a world leader, a monk, or a rabbi, or perhaps a recluse, or a housewife, or a businesswoman.

We are all born, certainly, with an array of skills and potentials – and with the free will to use them in constructive or destructive ways and manners. Perhaps these that come with us as parts of our body, or our mind, or our spirit, are seeking a kind of "hangover" effect from one life to another.

Children can be aided in developing their creative abilities if they can be allowed, in their early years, to express their memories of past lives as they see them in their more lucid moments – which often, to us, appear as moments when there is still sleep in their eyes, or when they are dreamy-eyed. For the creative parents, this can give an insight as to how to work with their children, for the betterment of both parent and child.

We have always had a close relationship with the Peter Riddle family here in Phoenix, the friendship dating back to India when Peter and I went to school together up to the mountain of Mussoorie, the foothills of the Himalayas. From the time our David was just a baby, there seemed to be a real bond relating him to Peter and Alice.

As David grew older, Alice frequently cared for him when Bill and I were away on trips. One morning, when he was four years old and Bill and I were eating breakfast, David came stumbling out of his bedroom, climbed up on my lap, with sleep still in his eyes and said, "Mommy, once when I was a black baby, Aunt Alice was my mommy." I tried to get more out of him, but the magic moment was gone.

It is sometimes difficult to piece together and find a pattern in the threads of one's past lives, if it does indeed exist. We've discovered that there seems to be a special purpose in living for each individual that one doesn't always realize, even though we may live all our lives searching for it.

The purpose of life here on earth suggested by the material in the Edgar Cayce readings is to grow spiritually. We could call this type of maturation process "soul growth." It is the growth that comes in spending many lifetimes striving to live in a creative, constructive manner.

A loving grandmother, who has spent much of her life in seeking for the meaning of that "soul growth" knew of my love for bringing new souls into the earth, and sent me the poem she fashioned in honor of her new unborn grandchild. It requires the honor of the printed page:

TO OUR NEW BABY

Here's to you, our baby new
So softly clothed in pink and blue –
Growing, learning every hour
In that same power that grows a flower –
And with you we must grow and learn
Since life's decree we must not spurn –
"For all Creation there is a goal –
Final perfection of this soul..."
So, we'll be not lost in wondering why

When turmoil comes to make us sigh –
But thank our Life at every turn
For another chance to live and learn.
And thus we may in wisdom say,
"Our privilege is to lead the way
That your new Life may know the gain
Of reaching heights we must attain."

Alice Shultz

It appears that too often we seek goals that are easy to find and are pleasurable, and not as centered in awaking our spiritual potential as they could be. As a result, it seems that we expend more and more energy uselessly, becoming more and more exhausted in the ruts we dig and the webs we've managed to tangle around ourselves.

It is then that the easy way becomes the hard way, for the law of cause and effect is always there for us to recognize and fulfill, and actions that are not constructive bring their own kind of results. To seek the difficult to achieve goals, on the other hand, the kind of activity that leads to creativity and helpfulness for others is often to find ourselves on a path that we classify as "hard." It may seem hard at first, but, because of the nature of the law, and because of the fact that we are "maturing" properly, the hard way becomes the easy way, and we find the bright path is our reward.

For the Hindu in the story of the World War I, his desire for peace brought him from a warlike nation to one that has fostered peace throughout its centuries of existence. He was granted his wish for an environment of peace, although none except himself could judge whether he really and actually feels peace inside – the kind of peace that comes from spiritual fulfillment of the soul's deepest desire.

Old wine in new wineskins? Maybe it isn't a farfetched idea. Maybe, when a baby is born, it is an opportunity for us to greet a soul who has much to share, much to experience, and who may help us as time goes on, much as we have greeted that one when he entered this sphere of experience.

CHAPTER THREE

The Baby Buggy

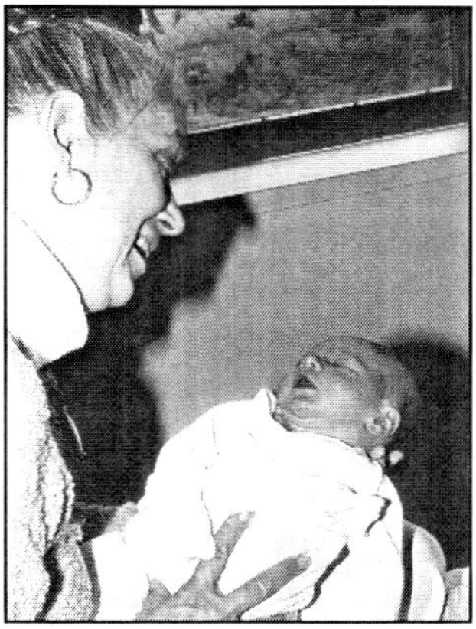

It was springtime in Missouri, and at Lee's Summit, Bill and I were scheduled to lecture on healing and birthing and lead a workshop on the same subject material. It was a program sponsored by the Association for Research and Enlightenment, and the site was the Unity Headquarters. It was 1972. There were about two hundred people there and the weekend moved rapidly.

During my last lecture, I was discussing the increasing frequency of home births that seemed to be happening all over the United States. I had seen it developing over the last few years and I had been called on to take care of postpartum problems when a husband or a friend had delivered a baby and things were not turning out right. I may or may not have seen the mother before that. It was a situation that no obstetrician wants or likes.

Suddenly, from somewhere out of my unconscious mind, I said, "What we need is a Baby Buggy, or a Delivery Wagon – a van that is equipped for emergencies and that can go out to the home when one of these women who wants a home delivery is about ready to have her baby. If we had such a vehicle and a nurse midwife to make it work, we would have met a need that is now not being met, and my belief system says to meet the needs of the condition."

Not much more was said at that moment, but after the lecture, several women approached me and talked excitedly about the possibility of us having a Baby Buggy at the ARE Clinic. I told them it would cost a lot of money, and one of the ladies handed me a check on the spot to get things started.

It took an extended incubation – or maybe the nine months humans wait for delivery of their baby does not apply to fully equipped vans for special purposes. Five years later, nevertheless, through gifts and the dedication of a lot of people, the Baby Buggy became a reality. It was equipped with all the "hardware" that is necessary to meet sudden emergencies that may come up during the delivery of the baby, and our nurse midwife, Barbara Brown, put the vehicle into full activity. It indeed met the needs of the condition – at least for a number of O.B. patients who desired to have their babies at home.

Our purpose in providing a home delivery program was not really to encourage families to have their babies at home, but rather to provide a viable alternative for those who for emotional, moral, or personal reasons choose to do so.

There are many people who feel that the place where a baby is born is a very special place. The Mohammedans still face "Mecca" when they pray because it was Mohammed's birth place. Joseph and Mary traveled all the way from Nazareth to Bethlehem so Jesus could be born, and then a cave or stable became a holy place because He was born there. The concept is that any place can become a holy place – a hospital, a cave, a taxi, a birthing room or center, or a home – depending on the attitude of the people involved.

The families involved in the home delivery felt that they wanted to spend time not just with the preparation of the mother's physical body during the pregnancy but also the preparation of the surroundings in which she labored and into which the baby would be born. They wished to have those people around who would contribute to a positive birthing experience and truly be a "welcoming committee."

There are many books written which talk about the importance of the mother being relaxed and not frightened. Fear is often the case in a strange environment such as the hospital delivery room, and certainly the mother is more comfortable in an environment which she has created. Our purpose here was not to go deeper into this aspect of the problem but to encourage families to do some in-depth consideration of what was right and good for them as they approached this most exciting, important event of their lives, so that the birth of their baby would be truly what it was meant to be – the bringing of divinity into materiality in a truly holy place and not just a happening.

In order to make the birthing experience as much of a growth experience as possible for all concerned, we asked the family to be involved in the program which prepared them and their home for the delivery.

Both parents-to-be began a five-week course, somewhere around the 30th or 32nd week of the pregnancy. It involved one evening per week for approximately two hours. During this "course" we explained the changes occurring anatomically, reviewed diet and nutrition, Caesarian section, mentioned the most commonly asked questions, introduced the importance of the "relaxation response" by practicing autogenics and the last two sessions were a brief review, with introduction and practice of breathing and exercises.

Surprisingly, belly dancing was included in the exercises. Over the years, I have wondered why a dance that involved so thoroughly the entire female body should be identified only with the belly. Further, I noticed that all the movements that the experienced belly dancer goes through are also those that are seen in the delivery of a baby; they involve the muscles of the lower abdomen and the perineum, and that would tend to loosen up and prepare the way for the parturition process.

This allows the mother to become aware right from the first trimester of the importance of her consciousness moving in her pelvis in such a way that the baby is not only enfolded in the physical comfort and protection of womb, but also emotionally and spiritually enfolded in love. She becomes aware of her bodily movements which enhance the baby's growth. By the time the baby is ready to be delivered, the mother's muscles are strong and mobile but also her tissues have been stretched and strengthened, her pelvis has become mobile so that the delivery itself is less painful and less traumatic.

The whole process of the belly dance as it is done and has been done for centuries, allows a baby who might be stuck in a certain position to be mobilized, moved and the position rotated by the movements of the mother's body and her pelvis. Rather than having to depend on a forceps for rotating a head that was stuck in a posterior position, the rhythmic movements of the mother's pelvis will allow that baby's head to be mobilized and the position shifted.

It's a sad state of affairs when we as physicians feel that we have to intervene during this natural process beyond what is necessary. I remember a number of years ago, having in attendance a young medical student from the University of Cincinnati. After the delivery was over, he said to me, "Thank you so much for letting me see this delivery. It's the first spontaneous delivery I've seen done without forceps." For me that was a shocking statement. To think that obstetrics was being taught in such a way that the intervention of forceps was considered the way of doing a spontaneous delivery!

Ann Clapp, who worked with the Edgar Cayce material, wrote an article about our Egyptian heritage. She found the following extract while surveying the Cayce readings about that country and their life styles:

> Q-7. Is there any particular type of dancing in which I should specialize in my teaching?
>
> A-7. Rather as we find, as indicated, there are two particular forms, the expression of the emotions for the BEAUTY of same; and that preparing the body for motherhood.
>
> Q-8. Would I be more successful by stressing my work with any particular group such as children – or adults exclusively?
>
> A-8. As might be drawn from just what is given; children in the expressive dance; adults – or the older – in their preparation for motherhood.
>
> For there are movements, there are portions of activities in dance which better fit for such than all the rubbings that may be given! 1626-1

Cayce's information was speaking about activities from thousands of years back, and we wonder just when that kind of thinking was active. The question may have been partly answered in the fall of 1979, when I saw a replica of an ancient Maya vase in a store window in Yucatan. The central figures depicted on the vase was a woman in obvious labor, about to have a baby and around her were several women dancing, dressed much as the belly dancer is seen to be dressed, and involved in much the same kind of a dance. So, from three worlds are found references of the belly dancer, one civilization bringing the ancient art into modern expression.

As we watched the girls in our program dance, we saw those who were near term became the graceful, beautiful dancers, and their bellies told the story.

Use of such a vehicle and the acceptance of home birthing as a viable alternative to hospital delivery brought into the Clinic a variety of patients who thought in terms of what might be called the "New Age." Shanti was one of these. Shanti was going to have a baby. She had done a lot of meditating and was adept at chanting. She understood much about the Spirit, but had some trouble relating to the material world around her. She went into labor early one morning.

When Barbara, our midwife, arrived at the home, the two of them worked together in the early stages of labor, with the breathing, but with not much success. Although she had had the prenatal classes teaching her about breathing with the labor contractions and instructing her about all the strange sensations she would be feeling, Shanti was just unable to get in touch with her body. She had real troubles relating to the progressing changes that came about in labor, and was painfully surprised at how the "labor pains" really hurt.

Barbara realized that Shanti's resistance to the physical changes was holding up the delivery and not allowing the cervix to open. Something had to be done which Shanti could understand and that would allow her to relax and bring about the normal progression of the birth process.

Shanti knew about meditation and knew that is one way of relaxing. But, she was not interested in meditating when it was hurting so much. Then, Barbara remembered that this young lady really liked to chant. And chanting is one way of getting rid of energy as well as balancing the body.

"Would you like to chant something, Shanti?" was her question.

"I'd love it, Barbara, but I'm hurting!"

"Never mind, Shanti, we'll think up a good chant for you and it will help take the hurt away and let you relax." Barbara was thinking fast. "Let's try this one, Shanti. You know the story about how the thousand pedaled lotus opens slowly to give enlightenment. Let's visualize that cervix as a lotus and lets chant, 'Open lotus, lotus open; open lotus, lotus open.' Let's try that and see what happens."

Shanti had not made progress at all up to that point. The cervix was dilated only about one centimeter. It took some time and a lot of chanting, but finally the lotus did open and the cervix was completely dilated; the head was ready to move down further into the birth canal, and it was time to push with the contractions.

Well, Shanti didn't want to push. Perhaps it would be better said that she didn't know how to push. The idea of working as she would with a bowel movement did not particularly entrance her. This was her baby. It wasn't just a daily task of emptying the bowels.

So, Barbara now had another problem. How was she going to get this girl to push? The chanting again seemed to be the answer, for Shanti certainly knew how to chant. What would it be this time? The lotus had already opened and this didn't seem to be in the present picture.

Barbara finally hit on it!

"Shanti, let's chant like this: 'Down and out; down and out; down and out.' That ought to get that baby moving. Let's try it."

Try it they did, and within an hour the baby was in its mother's arms, as she released tears of joy. The birthing organs were all in fine shape postpartum.

It was a lesson for the mother, certainly, but it was also the implementation of something that Barbara had known from way back – one must meet the person where she lives in consciousness, and it must be done in the midst of the living process, where we are, now.

Can you imagine the response of the hospital personnel if Shanti and her midwife or physician were to have let loose with that "Open lotus, lotus open" for five or six hours – not to mention the "Down and out" finale of the scene?

Use of our Baby Buggy allowed us to share in many other stories that dealt with the real unfolding of the real lotus within as more and more mothers found the home to be the place where they wanted to bring their babies into the world.

Barbara even did a delivery under a pyramid. Often a mother would labor through the first state on a waterbed and move to a firmer location on a beanbag for the actual delivery. But, whatever the place, it was one of the mother's choice and one where the attendant could work satisfactorily.

The Baby Buggy is no longer necessary since almost every hospital has its own birthing room where families are allowed to be part of the delivery process. Children, parents, grandparents and whoever is chosen as part of the welcoming committee are there allowing the mother to labor and deliver in a room properly equipped and beautifully designed for the specific purpose of making it a home-like environment and the delivery a more natural one.

CHAPTER FOUR

The Doctor's Responsibility

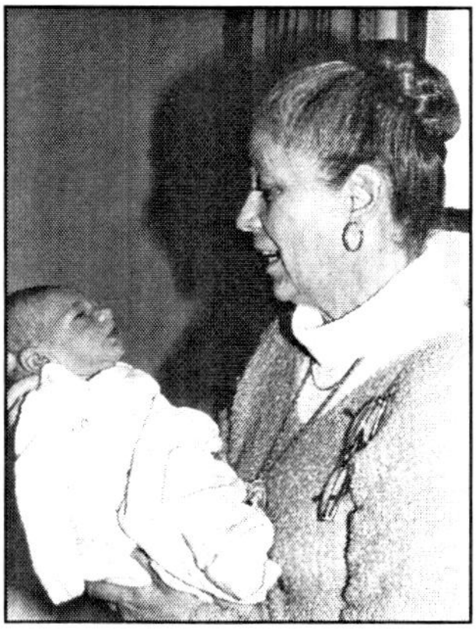

In ancient days, a physician was not just that – he/she was a physician-priest. He attended the physical body, certainly, but he was also the spiritual confessor, attentive to the needs of the mind and the spirit. For man has always been aware that he has a spiritual reality. Deep within his innermost parts, he has never lost that knowledge.

This kind of concept has always been an important part of my consciousness. I feel that if I don't extend my whole being to care for the whole being of the patient who has come to me for aid, then I am missing my calling. In caring for the woman who is going to have a baby, I cannot let that knowledge of caring lie dormant within me. I am called upon to be aware of the spiritual reality of the infant as yet unborn, and of the fact (as I see it) that this entity has come to restore relationships in the family where he is being born. There is an ongoing adventure here that must be shared.

My feelings on this score are shared by a multitude of other physicians, some of whom banded together in May, 1978, to form the American Holistic Medical Association.

Perhaps the time had arrived in the affairs of man that such ideals came to the fore among those who were actually out there practicing medicine. There have been individuals saying things like this from the time of Hippocrates.

The most lucid statement I have ever read challenging the physician to live up to the profession he has chosen is found in an essay, "To Be A Doctor," written by Dr. Felix Marti-Ibanez, now deceased. He was undoubtedly one of the outstanding medical writers. The essay was published and republished in M.D. magazine several years ago, and portions of it are certainly worthy of being reproduced here.

> To be a doctor, then, means much more than to dispense pills or to patch up or repair torn flesh and shattered minds. To be a doctor is to be an intermediary between man and god...
>
> Your duty to society is to be idealists, not hedonists; as physicians, to accept your profession as a service to mankind, not as a source of profit; as investigators, to seek the knowledge that will benefit your fellow beings; as clinicians, to alleviate pain and heal the sick; as teachers, to share and spread your knowledge and always because you are imbued with an ideal of service and not the ambition for gain. Thus, will you maintain the dignity of our profession as a social science applied to the welfare of mankind.
>
> Your duty to your patients will be to act toward them as you would wish them to act toward you: with kindness, with courtesy, with honesty. You must learn when and how to withhold the truth from your patients if by not telling them all the facts of the case you can relieve or console them, for you can cure them sometimes, and you can give them relief often, but hope you can give them always. Remember that a laboratory report is not an irrevocable sentence; behind all such reports and data, there is a human being in pain and anguish, to whom you must offer something more than an antibiotic, an injection, or a surgical aid; you must, with your attitude, your words and your actions, inspire confidence and faith and give understanding and consolation.[1]

Through the years I have been told that it is wrong to give a patient false hope. I don't think there is such a thing as false hope.

I think hope is a spiritual quality which is part of the whole healing process. By creating fear in the hearts of people we not only delay the healing, but often create a situation where healing cannot take place. We do not need to tell a patient untruths, but there is always something to hope for even in a terminal situation, for I truly believe that "hope springs eternal in the human heart."

Dr. Marti-Ibanez was talking about the role of the physician-priest. In spite of the possibility that most of us have forgotten the latter part of that role, perhaps we maintain that role in symbol form.

For, when we step into the delivery room, the first thing we do is change our clothes and don our gowns. We think the reason for changing is to maintain a sterile environment. The garments we wear are clean and sterile, and right for surgery or the delivery room. But, I wonder if that's the only function this ritual serves. Without realizing it, we may be symbolically donning those proverbial priestly robes.

Even without the gold braid and fancy decorations that may have been a part of the priestly robes of the past, the surgical gown may allow us to symbolize that role, while within ourselves we can consciously create that reality for the occasion, assuming our full posture as a physician-priest. Then we can bless the infant as he arrives, knowing that we, as part of the intermediary instruments between the divine and the material, can offer that blessing and know it will work.

We need to incorporate both roles, and the time has come for us to reawaken in our souls the knowledge that we hold a very special position.

Our daughter, Helene, was born knowing that she had to be a doctor. She identifies with the concepts of caring that Marti-Ibanez identified. But they developed at a later date than her conviction about being a physician. When she was just two years old, she came up to me one day and said, "Last time, when I was a doctor, I was a daddy doctor, not a mommy doctor." Well, this time she is a mommy doctor, and she probably has an earlier start than she did last time.

Helene was born with a purpose, and it's probably true that every soul is born with a purpose. But we don't consciously know what that purpose is. At least, most of us do not become consciously aware of it early in life. The time comes – a pinpoint of consciousness – when we become aware of that purpose, however, and when that happens, we are off and running, with an excellent chance of fulfilling what it was we came for.

Many years ago, before we were aware that we could influence the choice of vocation, of purpose in an unborn entity, I became pregnant with our first child. Carl was born the day after Christmas, but all through the later months of pregnancy we called him "Little Doc." It seemed only natural for us, since we were both physicians, and we couldn't think of a better way to spend one's life. So, our "Little Doc" grew – and when he was ready for his first Christmas, we have pictures of him with Bill's hat on his head and a stethoscope around his neck.

Well, Carl grew into manhood – a lot faster than I thought would happen – and he tried to avoid the field of medicine. He spent a couple of years in college majoring in fraternity and extra-curricular activities, but finally settled down. When faced with continuing in college or not, he said, "I can't imagine really doing anything except practicing medicine."

We both think Carl intended to be a physician before he was born, but we certainly programmed him early in life. I don't think he holds it against us, since we are still the best of friends. Today he is an orthopedic surgeon and loving every minute of it.

In the same way that we as parents helped Carl in his directions by visualizing what we thought he would become when he grew into adulthood, the physician can help the one who comes seeking help, whether it is a serious illness or a baby to be born. We can support that person in understanding the deeper meanings of life and help guide him toward a realization of the purposes that may be there to be recognized.

When we were in medical school we were told that it's important to treat your patients for their illness, to guide them in following a healthful diet and to get enough exercise. Nothing, however, was ever said about the kind of thoughts that one should be encouraging, nor the kind of books one should read, nor what kind of spiritual activity one might be involved in.

During pregnancy, all these have impact on the health of the mother and the kind of child that will be born. If a family wants to have a child that's in tune with the spirit and is going to bring more light and less darkness into the world, then I think that family had better spend a lot of time in prayer. Spiritual food is as essential to the purpose of the unborn infant as physical food.

If the mother is joyous and full of singing during the pregnancy, the baby is more apt to be a happy soul. On the other hand, the baby may influence the thoughts and feelings of the mother. If the two of them have had some disturbing times together in a past life, the mother may find herself laboring with some difficult feelings and wondering why.

A young physician friend of mine told me he had a patient in labor whose blood pressure began to rise. Instead of giving her medication to bring it down, he sat down and talked with her, relieving her anxieties and helping her to relax and laugh a bit. Much to everyone's surprise, she quieted down and the blood pressure normalized.

I had one girl who at eight months of pregnancy had her blood pressure moderately elevated. I became concerned and decided I would medicate her. She said she was a Christian Scientist and did not want medicine – she and her practitioner could get it down, she said. I agreed. After two weeks, her blood pressure was normal and she made it through the delivery without any trouble.

I have found that in women who are having trouble with elevated blood pressure, pre-eclampsia or even eclampsia, there is really an anxiety problem. The mother is often frightened or resentful (even if she isn't consciously aware of it). Often it is her first pregnancy and she is very unsure of herself, her position in life and certainly unsure of herself as a mother. Occasionally she is calm on the surface, but usually, with deep fears and often strong resentments. Resentment is an emotion which the mother is most ashamed to admit to herself, let alone anyone else. There is also the possibility that there is a deep-seated conflict in her being – part of her wanting the baby, part rejecting the newcomer and really frightened. All of these emotions are more intense and more difficult to deal with during a pregnancy.

Added to this is the fact that the relationships of all members of the family are being reawakened and reestablished. I have seen women who discover emotions foreign to their nature and experience, emotions they could not understand.

They have desires for foods and other stimulants which are not a part of their natural nature. I remember with my first pregnancy, I wanted green tomato pickles. I absolutely wanted green tomato pickles. It was right after the war and finding green tomato pickles was very hard but that's what I wanted. Any of my friends who came across a jar of green tomato pickles would get it for me and give it to me. With my second pregnancy, when friends of mine would find a jar of green tomato pickles they would get it for me and give it to me, and I could not stand green tomato pickles. It is interesting because my oldest son likes onions and garlic and food that is stimulating like that but my second son cannot eat them. So the question here is, whose desires were being fulfilled. It seems to me that I was a vehicle through which these two babies were fulfilling their own desires.

During my pregnancy with my fifth child, I ate peanuts. I couldn't get enough peanuts, trying to make them unsalted, but peanuts were top on my list. To this day whenever she comes into my home the first thing she does is go into my pantry to see if I have any peanuts.

Science has shown that taste buds make their first appearance in the fetus at eight weeks and are fully developed by the thirteenth week. By the fourteenth week, the hair-like microvilli cells that surround the taste buds complete the system. During this time in utero what they taste is the amniotic fluid which is the fluid that surrounds them throughout the pregnancy. They are constantly swallowing this fluid. In studies where different substances have been injected into the amniotic fluid, the babies response can be monitored.. It has been found that when the bitter tasting substances are injected, the babies stop drinking the amniotic fluid. However, if saccharin is injected, some babies increase their swallowing. Alcohol and nicotine seem to suppress the appetite. It is a well known fact now that mothers who consume alcohol and smoke have babies of lower weight and have a lower apgar score. This information, which is now available and accepted in scientific circles, validates what mothers who are sensitive have known through the ages.

Dr. Candace Pert in her groundbreaking book called *Molecules of Emotion* has carried this one step further in that she has identified particular hormones which fit particular receptors like keys fit locks. She has mapped the receptor sites for 50 or more neuropeptides (the amino acid compounds produced directly by nerve cells). These neuropeptides move up and down the nerve conduits within the brain and body and link three systems, the nervous system, the endocrine system and the immune system. Cells in the immune system are not only equipped with receptor sites for the neuropeptides, but they can manufacture the neuropeptides and other chemicals. These affect a person's emotions. They also make endorphins which are, in Dr. Pert's language, "the pleasure molecules." These pleasurable beta endorphins are found in the blood stream starting in the seventh week of pregnancy.

Now, if this sounds complicated, it is only because it is. Each family has its own set of circumstances and has to deal with them in their own way. We as physicians are fortunate for we can look into these living patterns and work with them. Instead of just medicating their bodies to overcome the toxemia and hyperemesis, we can allow our patients to talk about their dreams, their hopes, their fears, helping them overcome many of their problems.

As we watched patients' dreams, we began to understand that they were apparently picking up psychically the emotions and feelings of the incoming entity. The baby, of course, has feelings and emotions, residuals perhaps from an earlier incarnation.

I often asked the mother to try to make contact with the baby so she could get the energy or life force moving from where it was blocked at the level of the adrenal and move it up to the area of the thymus which is called the love center. I would have her record her dreams and see if she could contact the baby, also write letters to the baby telling him how she feels about things, and talk to him, trying to establish an early, helpful soul communication.

If the physician is not aware that something like this is going on, she will not be of a great deal of help in dispelling some of the difficulties that often arise in pregnancy. The physician is called upon to aid her patient with kindness, with gentleness, with honesty, and while giving hope to that person, also aid in understanding life's problems. In doing so, the physician may be saying, in a sense, to the woman who is about to have a baby, the same thing that Edgar Cayce said to one person who sought him out for a reading. She was also looking for the birth of a child:

> Let the body know, let the body comprehend that it is being chosen as a channel for the expression of divinity into materiality! 480-28

CHAPTER FIVE

Pregnant
To Be Or Not To Be

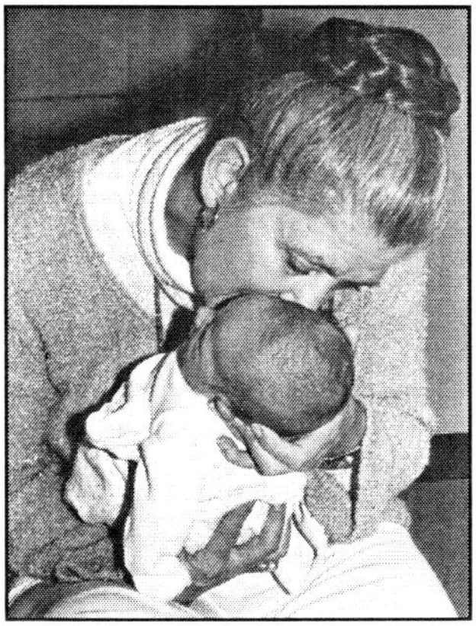

There are times when a would-be mother would give up all her possessions in order to become pregnant, but the odds just seem to be stacked against her. This was the kind of thing that happened to one of my patients several years ago.

Her tests at the hospital were inconclusive, she still didn't know why she could not become pregnant, and she was really low in spirits. She tells the story herself:

> In November of 1973, the night before Thanksgiving, I got out of the hospital after having some tests done. I was really low, lower than I ever remember being. I felt like I was carrying the weight of the world on my shoulders. When my husband was six hours late picking me up at the hospital and then dropped me off at a bowling alley for another three hours while he went back to work, I hit bottom. I am not a crier, but the inner sobbing was threatening to choke me.
>
> I was sitting in the restaurant which is separated from the bowling lanes by an open wrought iron wall. On the other side of the wall were two candy machines with about 18 inches of space between them.

Suddenly I became aware of a child standing there, about the size of two-year-old. There was a ceiling light shining on the child. I didn't know if the child was male or female because of the "different" haircut. I was surprised at how well the child spoke and was puzzled about its age. Dialogue as follows: (Remember, the child is looking at me through the wrought iron bars.)

Child: "You're in jail."

Me: "No, I'm not – you are!"

Child, looking around: "The whole world's in jail."

Me: "Who's going to let us out?"

Child, very matter-of-fact: "God will."

Me: "Who's going to ask Him for the key?"

Child, cocking his head to one side, thinking, then with a big joyful smile: "I'll ask God for the key to let you out."

At that instant, it was like a million pounds had been lifted from my shoulders – I was stunned by the freedom! Then I realized that the child was gone. I rose and went to look for the child, figuring that such a tiny child who spoke so well would be easily noticed. I could not find him – even asked several people if they'd seen him. None had! Then I began wondering if I'd had a vision.

Three years and three months later: I was having lunch at the same bowling alley with my son who was 28 months old. It was a very nice time. He was in the mood to talk quietly with mamma. Then he dropped his toy car through the bars and I went around to get it. When I stood up and looked at my son, he was watching me through the bars. He said, "Bless you, Mom," and instantly I realized that he was the child I saw three years before. He's very tiny for his age and speaks very, very well. And his haircut was exactly the same. Most people don't know whether he is a boy or girl at

> first sight. So you see, I saw my son two months before he was conceived.

Was there a key for the little boy to use to unlock the womb? The mother had been unable to get pregnant before that, and she was in the depths of despair. It seems to me that it is often just in this condition that one releases the hold on everything else, and can receive help. Her little son-to-be went to God and got the key which lifted her load and set her free. Perhaps the answer lies in the words spoken to another woman many years ago, as Cayce was giving help and comfort to her in a psychic reading:

> Q-1. Why has conception not taken place?
>
> A-1. Ask self! For, in the light of such as we have indicated, only in self may the answer come. Has God seen fit to give thee that thou seekest? Hast thou prepared thyself as a worthy channel of His consideration? Only self may answer.
>
> Q-2. Was there not enough time allowed before the menstruation.
>
> A-2. This is not a matter of purely a physical act. Do not consider same from the angle alone; else it will be to thine own undoing. 457-11

So, if we are to believe this woman's story, the information from the Cayce readings, and the Bible stories – such as the birth of the prophet Samuel to Hannah because of her prayers and her dedication of the hoped-for infant to the service of the Lord; if we are to believe these things, then pregnancy is not just a physical occurrence, but it is as Cayce described it to that same woman later on in that same reading – "although ovulation is a law of nature, conception is a law of God."

Sometimes the law of God becomes operative in strange ways. Friends of ours already had four children. The family had decided that four was enough, but, several years after the fourth arrived, the mother was taking a shower and she saw a blue light appear in the top corner of the shower.

Instinctively, she knew what the blue light meant. Another entity was wanting to make its appearance.

"Go away," she said, "You know I don't need any more kids!"

A month later, the blue light came back. Again the same dialogue. And again it happened. And again.

Finally, the reluctant mother gave in to the persistence of whatever the blue light meant, and she became pregnant. Child number five arrived, a boy, and her family was larger, and more complicated, of course, but more enjoyable.

Two years passed by. The mother of five had not ceased to take showers. The blue light came on once again. This time, she didn't have the energy to fight it any longer. It was almost as if she was getting a message from these two souls, as the blue light came on, that said, "Look, this is the place where I'm supposed to be. You are the people I am needing to live with, and this is the right time. So please get ready for me, cause I'm coming."

These things really happen. Perhaps I hear about them because I am willing to listen to these women who have feelings and experiences they don't want to have disregarded or made fun of. But they happen.

Another woman in writing to me told a similar story.

> During nursing school, I worked as a nursing tech part time. Occasionally, I worked a night shift, Unaccustomed to night work, I arranged to sleep at my friend's apartment during the time after the shift ended. While in a half dream sleep – I felt a white – blue warm light above my consciousness that entered me. I was alone when this happened. A month later, I missed my period and conceived Abraham.

Conception is one of the basic universal laws we don't really as yet understand. There is much more happening when the sperm and the ovum meet, and the electrical phenomenon occurs that marks the union of the two cells. It's not just a simple coming together, it is a meeting of many consciousnesses when a baby is conceived.

Conception is an instant in time when the soul who is to be born chooses where, when and why. It chooses the relationship between father and mother and itself. It sees what the environment for soul development may be in the family it is about to choose, and where there is a kind of unity of soul purposes, then there is the attraction. The choice is made, conception occurs and the process is begun.

It seems likely that babies do really choose their parents; only some, like the "blue light" babies, are more persistent than others.

I remember a time when I had two young mothers in my office at the same time. I went into the first room where a mother of four children was waiting for me. Two of the children were nursing at the same time. She was dressed in a long dress, her hair was in pigtails, and she had on no makeup. The children were happy, content and so was she. We dealt with whatever it was we were dealing with and I walked away from that room and into the next. Here I saw a young business woman with hair cut short, wearing high heels, neatly dressed in a suit, her makeup was flawless and her three year old son, whom I had delivered, was quietly playing target practice with a pencil on the end of a spring. We dealt with her problem and I went on.

I thought about these two women and how completely different their situations were, and how absolutely right each of the children were in the situation they had chosen. If I had taken the three year old from the business woman's family and put him into the other family it would have been a total misfit. She had to stop nursing him when he was two weeks old and she went back to work. If I had taken one of the children from the other family and put them into the business woman's family, they would have been totally lost. They just did not fit in each other's family situations but they really fit where they were. They were happy with their life choice and were dealing with life at its own level.

I call the first mother a marsupial mother because what she does so well and so comfortably is to keep her children clamoring around her all the time. Whereas the other mother would not be able to tolerate that and her child didn't need it and didn't want it.

If we listen to them, children will tell us their own story. This next little boy knew what he wanted.

> After telling my three year old son, Christian,
> "I love you so much, I'm so glad God gave me you,"
> he replied, "Yea, and she gave me to someone else

> and I said, 'No, that's not the one,' and then she gave me to you, Mommy. Then I said, 'Yes, that's the one!'"

There are many methods of contraception. None of them absolute in their effectiveness unless surgery is employed. Several years ago, one of my patients was fitted with an I.U.D., an intra-uterine device. They had enough children, and this was a considered move to prevent any more being added to the family.

The husband, in the course of his business, was required to make regular annual trips to Hawaii. On one of his trips, however, he had a disturbing dream. In the dream, he was in Hawaii with his wife and their two children, aged 10 and 12. A man dressed in white approached him in the hotel lobby, smiled gently at him and handed him an I.U.D. "Your wife is pregnant, sir!" The man then disappeared and the dream ended.

Although the dream was a bit disturbing, he and his wife discussed it and discarded it's obvious message because she did have the device in place and it had worked for these past six years.

In the spring, his work piled up more than he had anticipated, and he felt it was best to cancel the trip to Hawaii. The weeks passed by, and his wife confided to him that her periods had stopped. A visit to our office, and I told them that she was pregnant despite the I.U.D.

When the time arrived for delivery, everything went smoothly, there were no complications, the labor was short and the I.U.D was delivered before the baby. After I removed the device I turned around to face the husband, who by now was grinning a bit. I handed him the I.U.D., just like in the dream, and I gently said, "Your wife is pregnant, sir!" By that time both the mother and the dad knew this entity who had come into the family, and they were giving her a royal welcome. Oh yes, my gown was white.

Husbands are not only involved in dreaming about their wives and pregnancy, but they can also participate in morning sickness. In the July 1978 issue of the *American Journal of Maternal Child Nursing*, Dr. Jacqueline Fawcett, R.N., of the University of Connecticut describes research involving men who respond to their wives' pregnancies in strange ways. Regardless of their culture – even here in the United States – men sometimes experience sensations of the body-image changes in keeping with their wives' pregnancy. The body is not altered although the body-image is. The husbands experience increased or decreased appetites, gastrointestinal upsets, nausea and vomiting, fainting, leg cramps, backache, and all the rest of those things usually associated with pregnancy.

In the South Pacific, an ancient practice called couvade is followed by the men of the villages whose wives are pregnant. They have these same symptoms, take to bed and even imitate her bodily movements during labor. The symptoms are believed to be an expression of the husband's involvement in the pregnancy and his identification with his wife.

Dr. Fawcett did not report, however, on any cases similar to one that crossed my path of experience well over forty years ago. A young woman, whose husband had been shipped out to Korea almost immediately after they were married, came into my office and was worried about her health. It didn't take a great deal of medical diagnostic ability for me to tell her she was pregnant. She was unable to contact her husband until she heard from him three months later.

It seems that when he arrived in Korea, he had been afflicted with severe nausea, and it continued even after he was placed in sick bay. Every morning he would vomit, and he continued to be quite ill most of the day – was unable to go back to duty. The medication given would afford him temporary relief. Lab tests and x-rays revealed nothing of significance. His gastrointestinal tract was all right.

The problem continued until he received a letter from his wife telling him that she was pregnant. The medics treated him for morning sickness, and his symptoms finally cleared up after the first trimester of his wife's pregnancy.

A beautiful letter from another father tells the same story:

> My daughter, was born 1/8/72. Our first child. During the 70's I was a traveling salesman. My wife was very pessimistic that I would be on the "road" when our child was born. I kept telling her, "No I'll be home." The summer before our child's birth, my wife and I kept trying to agree on a name. We couldn't agree!!! What to name the child if a

boy; what to name the child if a girl????? This was getting ridiculous!

We went to sleep one night. I slept well and woke the next morning with a name in mind. I have no conscious recollection of communicating with our unborn baby but I woke knowing "it" would be a girl and her name is Mona. My wife liked the name and agreed, if the baby was a girl.

Due date was last week of January. Every other week I left home Tuesday and returned Thursday afternoon. We live in Sacramento, California, and I traveled to Reno and Lake Tahoe. I was going to make one more trip before the due date. I usually finished a trip early in the afternoon and got home three or four hours later, this trip I didn't finish till 5:30 PM. I was very tired, hungry and could see snow clouds over the mountains. I was in Reno. I telephoned my wife to see how she was feeling and tell her why I was so late. She felt fine and we agreed I should stay in Reno and leave early the next day.

As I say, I was real tired and quite hungry, My dinner was half eaten when I got up from the table, went back to my motel, packed up and started home. As I got up from the table in the restaurant I asked myself, "What are you doing?" I could see that it was snowing in the mountains and I really don't like to drive in the snow. Three hours to drive home and I WAS BEAT.

I arrived home about 10 PM. My wife was quite surprised to see me and asked what caused me to change my mind and drive through a snow storm when I was soo tired? I said "I don't know but I JUST couldn't resist the urge to come home." We drank a cup of coffee and went to bed.

My wife woke at midnight and said the baby was on its way! Mona was born at 4:30 am. As the nurse brought her out and showed her to me, I looked at her and said, "Hi, it's been a long time." The nurse

> looked at me like I was crazy. I felt so dumb! Why would I say something like that?
>
> That night in Reno, Nevada, I COULD NOT RESIST THE URGE TO COME HOME! Now if that wasn't Mona telling me come home because she was going to be born that night and I promised to be there, then what was prompting me?
>
> The last thing I wanted to do was drive through a snow storm late at night, tired and hungry! But I did! Sure glad I did too!!!

Isn't it interesting how the connection between individuals can reach over thousands of miles when the concern and love are of such a nature that certain firm relationships are established?

A Cayce reading adds depth and affirmation to such an idea:

> ...Each experience builds the ability of the individual, either mentally, spiritually or physically, to make application in whatever may be the next experience. And in this relationship, remember that opportunity arises with each meeting, each association. Each problem has its opportunity for choice of spiritual, mental, material opportunities. They are one in their greater, their better sense. 2489-1

So it would seem that a series of lifetimes would afford a woman to experience times when it would be advisable and constructive to have children, and other periods when it would not. Each could be a helpful, creative experience, physically, mentally, and spiritually.

CHAPTER SIX

New Light On Abortion

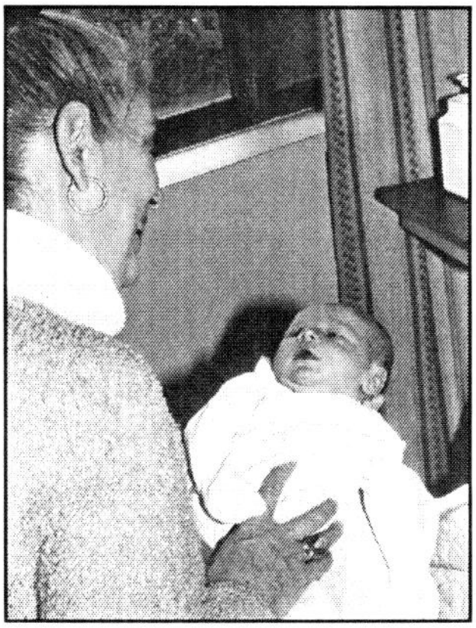

Abortion has been a topic always explosive in nature as the pros and cons of the subject come into view. I have had a great deal of difficulty in trying to come to some sensible conclusions about the problem. The spontaneous abortion is no real psychological or ethical tug-of-war, but when it comes to an induced end to a pregnancy, there are literally thousands of well meaning men and women on both sides of the dividing line, and I was torn between the two warring factions.

As the concept of the continuity of life grew in its reality in my mind, and the pieces started to fall into place – how we have no beginning and no end as spiritual creatures; how we choose our parents; how we may see what lies ahead, no matter what it may be; how experiences are for our growth and understanding – I began to feel a bit better about abortion when it was really needed. The idea of reincarnation helped.

But I still had a problem with women who wanted an abortion because it was convenient, or because the pregnancy was embarrassing or threatening the stability of a marriage. These things didn't make sense to me – I always adhered to the principle of sticking to something I had started.

I suppose my long familiarity with the Bible story and my 45 years of working with the Cayce material gave me much food for thought. The following reading seemed to be saying to me that there is purpose in everything that comes as an experience in life, but I'm not sure I really understood it in its full implications:

> For, in the comprehension of no time, no space, no beginning, no end, there may be the glimpse of what simple transition or birth into the material is; as passing through the other door into another consciousness.
>
> Death in the material plane is passing through the outer door into a consciousness in the material activities that partakes of what the entity, or soul, has done with its spiritual truth in its manifestations in the other sphere. 5749-3

One day, however, a new day dawned in my consciousness. The business of abortion became more understandable. Not that I would have an abortion myself, in my present level of awareness, but I can see that it is frequently reasonable, understandable, and the "right" thing for a woman to do. (We won't get into that definition of "right.") The new light dawned with a story one of my patients told me some time ago.

This mother had a four-year-old daughter whom she would take out to lunch occasionally. They were talking about this thing and that, and the child would shift from one subject to another, when Dorothy suddenly said, "The last time I was a little girl, I had a different mommy!" and she started talking in a different language. Her mother quickly retrieved a pencil from her purse and copied down what her daughter had said as nearly as she could understand it. (In the meantime, she has lost the piece of paper.)

The magic moment seemed over, but then Dorothy continued, "But that wasn't the last time. Last time when I was four inches long and in your tummy, Daddy wasn't ready to marry you yet, so I went away. But then, I came back." Her eyes lost that faraway look, and she was chatting again about four-year-old matters.

Mother was silent. No one but her husband, the doctor and she knew this, but she had become pregnant about two years before she and her husband were ready to get married. When she was four months pregnant, she decided to have an abortion. She was ready to have the child but her husband-to-be was not.

When the two of them did get married and were ready to have their first child, the same entity made its appearance. The little child was saying in effect, "I don't hold any resentments towards you for having had the abortion. I understood. I knew why it was done, and that's okay. So here I am again. It was an experience. I learned from it and you learned from it, so now, let's get on with the business of life."

Maybe the child didn't have that kind of vocabulary, but that was in essence what was being said, and what was being related to the mother. It does throw a new light on abortion, doesn't it? Every experience is for the individuals involved, and all abortions do not have this kind of circumstance surrounding them, naturally, but I could see how things were different than I at first thought.

An interesting addition to this 1977 story came in a letter I received from her in 1982. Her daughter who had given us this insight into abortion was now 16 and her mother's letter to me includes the following account:

> In November of 1979, my daughter came to me and said she was pregnant. We both menstruated on the first of the month. I did and she didn't. My husband and I talked and meditated about it and felt in our heart of hearts we could (if it was my daughter's wish) accept and love the child into our family. We wanted to give her an alternative to abortion. The decision had to be hers and she decided on November 28 to abort. Well, the next week I didn't have a period, but had a dream. (You will remember that in December, 1977, I had abdominal surgery and had sections of both tubes removed to prevent pregnancy).
>
> The dream: "I saw an infant being carried out to sea on the top of a wave. I ran after it into the surf scooped it up in arms and brought it onto the sand, the color blue was around."
>
> A week later I had a pregnancy test which was positive. Needless to say, my husband and I were in a state of shock; it was like an altered state of consciousness.

This story is truly amazing to me since apparently the little boy who was not going to be born to the 16 year old daughter still wanted to be part of the family and in spite of the fact that the grandmother had a tubal ligation, he found his way into the family and was born. This is one of those wonderful stories that makes me truly understand that life and love have dimensions that we cannot even begin to comprehend let alone control.

If the entity really understands what is happening, if there is a reality to consciousness in all spheres of life, and if a couple makes the decision to have an abortion in an understanding, thoughtful manner – with the feeling that somehow this is really the right thing to do – then somehow, I think, there is communication with the Divine, and the outcome is bound to be a constructive, learning event.

The mother's story really did something for my understanding – it provided me with another dimension from which to think out the solution to the problem when I'm working with patients who are considering an abortion.

A 15-year-old girl came to the Clinic one day, pregnant and distraught. She was still a child, really, not ready to have a baby. She reminded me of a patient Bill had back in Wellsville, who became pregnant at 11. It was difficult forty-five years ago to get an abortion, but the girl managed it in a nearby town and we thought that was the best thing to do.

This pregnant girl, just 15, and her family were all confused about what should be done. I suggested to them that they make a decision, pray about it, ask for dreams, and then let me see them again after they had come to a firm conclusion.

The return visit revealed that they had all come to the same decision – there should be an abortion. They all felt that it was the best thing to do. I began the arrangements to have it done, but the next morning I got a call from the family – the girl had aborted spontaneously. I checked her in the office and all was well.

Did the entity that was scheduled to come in get in on those plans and considerations that the family was making? One never knows when the curtain falls finally on a drama such as this, but it makes one wonder. Perhaps that individual is in a holding pattern until the girl is ready to have her first child. Perhaps, on the other hand, the experience was what was needed, and that particular entity will find what is needed elsewhere.

The story has fascinating implications. Perhaps there is a spontaneous release mechanism that comes into operation when all the questions are faced with depth of insight, with prayer and with communication with the Divine within, and induced abortion then is not necessary.

I've known several other girls who have had the same type of life-changing experience in the years since this first event came about. When the lesson is learned, when the person understands what needs to be done, then life itself – we call it nature – takes over and changes the course of events, and a spontaneous abortion is the result.

When one of these situations arises now, I ask the young woman to take time to write down all of her reasons and feelings for having an abortion and the reasons and feelings against having an abortion. Then, in as unemotional a way as possible, make the best decision she can make for all concerned. Then prayerfully go on about the business of life, either getting the abortion done or not. The next three women tell a similar story.

> 1981. I thought I was pregnant and very upset about the possibility. That night at home sitting on the couch I forced myself to calm down. Finally, able to reach a meditative state I began a dialogue with the entity as if it were there beside me. Talking honestly of the situation and asking that with love it could release me. Suddenly, I wasn't pretending anymore. I had the absolute certainty that the entity was not next to me on the couch, but over to the right and a foot or so toward the front. We engaged in a very emotional dialogue. Out of the corner of my eye when I didn't try to focus on the area I saw something there, an undefined mass, but a mass of consciousness with feelings and needs.
>
> Exhausted from crying and on totally new ground with the experience of meeting the entity that was growing a vehicle inside of me, I went to

bed. Throughout most of the night, I surrounded the entity and myself with love, but kept firmly stating that I was not the proper receptacle and it must release me.

The next day at 11:00 A.M. I called the father of this child to tell him I was pregnant and working to release the entity. He was shocked by the pregnancy news and totally retreated. I felt abandoned. One hour later a searing pain shot through me; 10 minutes after that I began to bleed; and 8 hours later the actual miscarriage occurred amid tears of release as well as deep sadness. (I always wanted a child.)

I was 3-1/2 months pregnant and our family life was a total disaster! I could not do anything right for my husband, our daughter of 2-1/2 was an irritation to him, he worked or fished or was with his friends, but always angry at home and blaming, etc. I did not know he was alcoholic. But one day during an ongoing tantrum that started at 8 A.M. I had finally had enough. As he was still yelling at me at 2 A.M. I became very quiet within myself and asked God and this child to not be pregnant any longer. I explained I did not know what was wrong with this family but no one should come into this unhappiness. I felt I did not have strength to care for him. I had a responsibility to my family and was afraid of what was becoming of us. I asked that if he needed to come, to understand the situation and my lack of ability to care for him as I felt was right. Three days later I miscarried. I returned home with an extremely deep commitment to pull this family together and with much gratitude for the child I'd just lost. I wished him well and hoped it had provided him with an experience that he needed and if he wished to come again when the family was more united that it would be fine with me. I experienced grace and set out to do my best.

I began to admit to the fear of alcoholism and our lives took a very new road – slowly, after that.

When I realized I was pregnant, I talked to my most loving friend and teacher. She mentioned that maybe I should speak to the entity or at least 'tune in' and get a feel for the entity.

I pondered this thought for at least a week and one night I decided, OK what did I have to lose? Nothing but an unwanted pregnancy! So for a week I began thinking about this entity who came into my life and wondering about the entity and began slowly to pop out questions like why are you here? Why would you want to come to this family now? What do you need and what do I need from you?

Inside a week, I was looking closely at my marriage and with a much different looking glass. I began to actually thank this entity for helping me to see clearly where I needed changes in my marriage and my approach to child rearing. It was a wonderful growing experience. Then one night I decided to talk to this entity who I now felt very close to and began to watch my emotions and feelings change about the pregnancy. I realized the issue was not the pregnancy but rather my marital differences. I felt a wonderful rapport with this entity who I was sure would incarnate as a female; she was very special to me and my emotions ran away with me and I felt that I began to actually know this entity. I decided to make a pro and con list of the pregnancy, the con list was loaded with reasons why not to have a second child. The pro list had only one, a playmate for my son. When I looked at the list I stared for quite some time since I was in a state of disbelief I could not understand why I could not find 1 or 2 more reasons to have this child.

Well, the confusion was gone, within a week I spoke again to the entity and together we decided against using this vehicle at this time – it was a

> mutual decision and we parted with a deep love and understanding for each other. Within one week I began spotting and the pregnancy aborted itself – Miraculous Indeed!

It has surprised me how many of the girls, after going through this process, have decided to keep the pregnancy.

I now always tell the mother to communicate with the entity who is hovering, waiting to be born. "Tell that individual what is happening, and why it is happening. This makes things more in accord with life patterns and needs for all those involved." I've wondered if this is what happened in the story that was given to me recently by one of my patients:

> Several years ago, I was about sixteen days pregnant, unexpectedly, when I was closely exposed to German measles. To make a long story short, the baby, Grey Andrew, was born in due time, apparently normal. He was not, however, and died at two weeks of age, with two abnormal openings to his heart.
>
> About four years after that, we finally had another child, a girl. Then fifteen months later, after another unexpected pregnancy, Rowan was born. I always felt Rowan was the same soul entity as Grey Andrew but never said anything, because there was no evidence to suspect this, or to support it.
>
> A few months ago, my 24 year-old-son, Carroll, came to me and said, "Mom, I had the oddest dream. For what it's worth, this soul entity came to me, saying it was the same entity that had been Grey Andrew, and was now Rowan."
>
> Carroll asked the entity why he hadn't stayed on as Grey Andrew. The entity replied that he hadn't felt able to accomplish what he had to at that time. Carroll was a little skeptical, in the dream, and the entity said, "Well, if you need a little more convincing – notice the similarity in our birth dates – notice the threes."

> Grey Andrew was born December 3, 1963 (12/3).
>
> Rowan was born February 13, 1968 (2/13).
>
> Both 1, 2, 3. (I'm convinced!)

Then early in 1978, a woman who was attending our annual medical symposium gave me a letter that she had written about her experience with pregnancy and abortion. This is her story:

> I've had three pregnancies, and have two girls, 15 and 11. I was on the birth control pill after Ann was born for about a year and decided to stop the pill and have a second child. It took almost a year to get pregnant. During the second month of pregnancy, I slipped and sat down hard on a messy cement ramp. Felt fine, but from that time on the fetus did not develop. The doctor questioned his original diagnosis and said I probably was not pregnant. I went almost to five months before I aborted. Although it was spontaneous and clean, I had a bad infection.
>
> About four months later, I became pregnant with Mary. Unlike the preceding pregnancy, I felt great – pregnancy does agree with me – I'm a Cancerian. The L & D (labor and delivery) was normal; she weighed 9 pounds 9 ounces. Hoping for a boy, I thoroughly expected to be disappointed when I had a girl. When they laid her on my tummy, however, I knew her and became so excited, and began talking to her saying things like, "I didn't know they would let you be my baby." I have always thought since, that she had once been my "invisible" playmate, my "little sister."
>
> Last year, while driving home from Asilomar with Ann and Mary, we started talking about how they were born and their early days. As I finished Mary's story for her she was quiet for a while. I thought she had fallen asleep.
>
> Suddenly, she blurted out, "I killed it."

> My reaction was, "Killed what?"
> "Your baby, Mama."
> "No, honey, I fell, remember?"
> She said, "No. It was a boy and I wanted to be a girl!" This shut me up. She is normally a very feeling little girl – it struck me that she said it in such a matter-of-fact way I was anxious if this was so that she would not feel guilty about it. I tried to reassure her, but she did not seem to understand or need it. It was a fact to her, not like a death at all.

The next story tells us how aware the mother and baby can be about each other:

> I am 51 years old. At 34 years of age, I conceived my third child, already having two children, ages six and ten. From the moment of conception, I was uncomfortable with it. It was not a planned child, and I tried to become happy with the event, but could do nothing but cry for four months. I have a good marriage and two beautiful children and my husband was very supportive of the pregnancy, and so it should have been right. At four and one-half months for no apparent reason, my fetus aborted. When the baby decided to leave me, and I knew at the exact moment because the fetus felt lifeless or loose, that we never had a close association, and to this day I believe I mentally, but not deliberately aborted the fetus. The gynecologist at the hospital had no explanation for this miscarriage and said the fetus appeared to be fine.

I wonder if life could have been different for a mother who wrote to me just recently if she had been able to explain her situation to her son before she had her abortion. Let me share her letter with you.

> My son, age 13, became deaf as an infant and has been extremely violent with me and others, over all his young years. So much so, he does not

live with me now. I had the privilege of listening to two of your tapes. While listening to them my mind began to work with little assistance from me, slowly at first, then with such accuracy and speed, pieces started fitting about my son and myself, until I felt quite dizzy with realization. I wrote everything down as quickly as I could. It then became clear to me why my son has been so angry. He had been trying to be born of me, since 1949, if not sooner.

My friend suggested I write to you as these are astonishing facts, to me, and he felt you may be able to offer me some assistance, or anyway share these facts with me.

The facts are:

1. In 1949, thirty years ago, I became pregnant by rape and had a voluntary abortion performed when I was approximately 5-1/2 weeks pregnant. Four years later, married, I did give birth to a daughter.

2. When she was three, in 1956 (7 years after my first pregnancy), I became pregnant again in a tube, which, when removed was said by the surgeon to be 5-1/2 weeks "pregnant."

3. In 1963 (again, 7 years later) I had what the doctor termed a false pregnancy – not a miscarriage even – a "false pregnancy." After having cysts removed from the uterus and vaginal area, plus a D & C performed on me, I was told I would be unable to become pregnant again. (For years I was determined to have three children.)

In 1965, we adopted a child at birth, sight unseen. (Here I will recall for you when I learned of this soon-to-be-born child, through my doctor, I was hysterical for three days when my husband told me we could not adopt another child. I told him it would be as if I was refusing my own blood son and my husband finally relented and we did adopt my boy.)

When he, my son, was 5-1/2 weeks old, he contracted strep infection and double pneumonia, was hospitalized, and nearly expired two times his first day there. Over a period of eighteen days he received more than one hundred injections of streptomycin to save his life. At three months of age, I was certain he was deaf and this was confirmed when he was seven months old. His extreme anger began early.

When he, Phillip, was six and a half or seven years of age, his violence began, seemingly as much to his surprise now and then as to me and others.

No one can ever make me believe differently now if I was to tell anyone but you and those I know from the energy circle. My son finally found his way to me through adoption, in extreme anger. Possibly he was a dominant figure for me in our other lives – he has unfinished business. Now, recalling actions and words he has spoken to me help make it even more clear.

"I was supposed to be here first."

"Why didn't you want me first."

"You were bad to me – you wanted my sisters first."

He has said these words and others to me over the years, which meant no more to me than his ego was hurt because he is the youngest. When I did send him away from me to live with others, he told me then and since, that he would be "finished" being angry with me when he is fourteen and "I can come to live with you then, Mom." I now believe this. A new seven year cycle and our opportunity to bring our lives together. I can help now. He has always known! I just found out. I will see him for a nine day spring holiday in another week. I recently spoke with him over the phone and his speech has improved greatly. Whether it is his ability or my ears – his speech is clearer to me.

I would like to hear from you, Dr. I am sorry I do not remember your last name, Dr. Gladys, but am sure this letter will find its way to you.

> I have so much to do now and am hoping I will be guided well.

Is abortion, then, something to take lightly? It would seem from these stories – all of them real living experiences – that the important thread holding them all together is the nature of consciousness found in those who are faced with the big decision. If there is communication, if there is prayer, if there is sought understanding of a life purpose – or at least the direction toward a life purpose – and if there is the awareness of the continuity of life and the reality of choices each person can make that are either constructive or destructive, then when the choice is made, it will be right for that time and place. Those who have fulfilled prerequisites like these may indeed have thrown new light on abortions.

CHAPTER SEVEN

More About Abortion

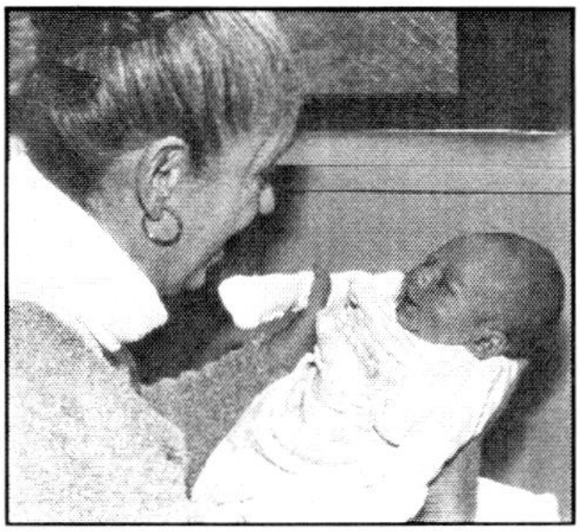

The question of abortion is extremely complicated and I believe when we try to oversimplify it into issues that are either right or wrong we frequently miss the underlying human values which deal with true compassion and caring. If we get so focused on either the baby or the mother and make judgments which come solely from our own experience and our own philosophical background we may find ourselves in positions with lack of understanding. We may be dealing with issues which have little to do with God's love and caring presence.

A number of years ago I had a patient I had cared for for many years. She was one of these women who had been unwell all of her life. It was as if her constitution had trouble dealing with life's issues. So when she found out she was pregnant at age forty, she and her husband had to make some very difficult decisions. After a great deal of prayer and counseling, and work with her inner being, they decided that they would go ahead and have this baby. Once this decision was made, they were extremely happy and prepared for the new arrival. When she was almost three months pregnant they had an ultrasound done and found that the baby was severely defective. He had many congenital anomalies and would probably be unable to function in this dimension even if he was carried to term. With that information they had to reexamine the position they had taken. Again with deep soul searching and prayer they decided that where they might be able to deal with and raise a "normal" baby they simply could not see carrying the added load of a baby that had this many problems. So with deep grief and pain she went ahead and had the abortion. When she came home after the abortion, her phone was ringing. She picked up the phone and a woman from her prayer group screamed over the telephone, "Murderer!" That experience was so traumatic for her that she has never truly recovered from it. It was a time of deep vulnerability when she was wide open to emotional responses and reactions and when a woman who she considered a friend and prayer partner condemned her with such vehemence, it literally shattered her spirit. I believe that the lady who screamed "Murderer" at her friend probably traumatized the soul and spirit of her friend as severely as the mother who had the abortion did to the fetus that was coming.

I believe that it is our place to support each other in times of crisis, whether we agree with each other or not. When we do not help each other we are adding to the pain and suffering of the world, not helping it.

The next story comes from a women who had struggled very deeply with the pain of having had an abortion done and in the process communicated with the unborn baby and has written a touching story. The pain that she and the unborn baby suffered is clearly manifested in her words that follow:

> My experience in my abortion was one of the most intense periods of spiritual growth in my life. I believe it was for the spirit too. Death and Birth seemed to lose all meaning or meant the same. For a while I felt Oneness with the spirit child. Enclosed is a poem I wrote and a piece of writing that came into my mind and quieted me after the abortion. I felt closer and more loved and at one with God during this painful period than I ever have in my life. I received much inner reassurance that I did the loving act for all concerned.
>
> "The plastic stick turned blue, me too, I crumbled, 15 years ago another positive result had me on top of a rock crying, – a marriage proposal, fear,

acceptance, a husband in Nam, a pregnancy, a baby girl, wonder, joy, a bug ridden apt. in Calif, isolation, a house, another positive result, a baby boy, joy, wonder, laughing busy, playing busy, cleaning busy but whispers, whispers, whispers in my head. Don't let it happen to them. Don't let it happen again, (pain, isolation) I hurt I hurt I hurt I hurt. Daddy Heart attack. Fear, don't leave me here. How will I see me without your eyes Headaches, Headaches, Headaches, vision impaired, blacker, blacker being born into a universal Love all in the same instant was an awfully painful trauma. God, as some of you call Her or Him, whichever you prefer, has been taking care of that pain by helping me learn about my human nature. I'm pretty well over the anger and hurt I felt when I first got here. Right now I'm having another problem. I decided to write you about it.

I feel very miserable about the anger and hate my conception and termination has caused. It hurts like crazy to think that my existence as a human soul is causing all this destructive horrible behavior among you. I'd like to try and help.

I'm beginning to see that there is unbornness in all of you too. As a matter of fact, that's why my mother aborted me, unbornness. She loved me. She cried for weeks before and after her decision. She spends time every day mourning me, wondering about me. Not many of you had shown her much kindness or care. She was hurt and tired inside. She felt aborted herself. She didn't trust herself or the world to give me what I needed to grow. So I am here, instead of with you on earth.

Some of you call her a murderer. Who do you think she is...God? Human souls can't endure unlimited amounts of neglect and hate and still be healthy enough to care for ME! How can I believe you are able to love me when you gave her spirit such a beating? You terrified me a lot by doing that.

Some of us unborn think that those of you who insist on our birth, no matter what the circumstances, are treating us and our mothers like livestock. What are you doing to make sure we are getting the love and care we need to feel human after we're born? Quite a few of us would have spent a lifetime never feeling we were needed or lived or even human until our deaths or suicides. Oh yes, there are a lot of those souls here too. The ones who wished they'd never been born and then aborted themselves. They often say they are jealous of us and wish their mothers had taken the responsibility and aborted them in the beginning. It takes Love or God, whichever you prefer, a lot longer to heal those who endured living abortions. You know who I'm talking about, people exposed to rejection, abuse, and neglect, until they felt less than human. Your mental institutions and prisons are full of them. Others walk the streets alone, cry alone, eat alone, and find no joy or love in being a part of the human race. You try hard to love, but millions still exist as tormented living abortions. Just look at the countries where there's not even shelter or food for me. Sometimes the world seems as limited as my mom in being able to care for me.

I am not really fragile at all, in fact as a human spirit I am quite indestructible. This makes me subject to an inhuman amount of pain because I am also sensitive and vulnerable to others, and easily aborted in a number of ways. I realize now that I had a lot to offer the world with my birth, but sometimes I get angry and scared thinking about what you had to offer me. Take those living abortions I was talking about, they have as much to offer as I did. It strikes me as quite spoiled of you to spend so much of your time and energy fighting for my physical existence. When I look at all the human souls that have already been wasted I think… If I had been born, and that had happened to me, I wouldn't be feeling human now, I'd be alive and feeling like trash. I'm just as angry at you about those abortions as you are at my mother for aborting me.

There are millions of us here, all for different reasons. We are here because of maternal instinct you left unborn or aborted in our mothers. We are here because we were conceived in the violence of rape. We are here because our mothers were children themselves and our arrival could have further aborted our souls and theirs'. We are here because our mothers had been living in aborted agony for years and needed to give themselves the nurturing they never received from others. More and more of us are here being spared the pain filled reality of a hopelessly deformed or diseased physical existence. We are here because we had mothers who recognized that they, as humans, were limited, and had no emotional, financial or physical space left for us. We are here because of the physical and emotional, limits and realities, inherent in being human.

I appreciate the grief some of you feel in losing me, but your anger at my mother hurts, and makes me feel ignored. To give birth to a human soul takes only a moment, to give that soul a full and loving human experience is a precious but difficult lifelong responsibility, and trust. It is a responsibility that can never be met by those unwilling to meet it. It cannot be forced on those unable to accept it. I am sad I did not get to live, I miss my Mommy. I wish she hadn't been aborted."

CHAPTER EIGHT

Dreams In Pregnancy

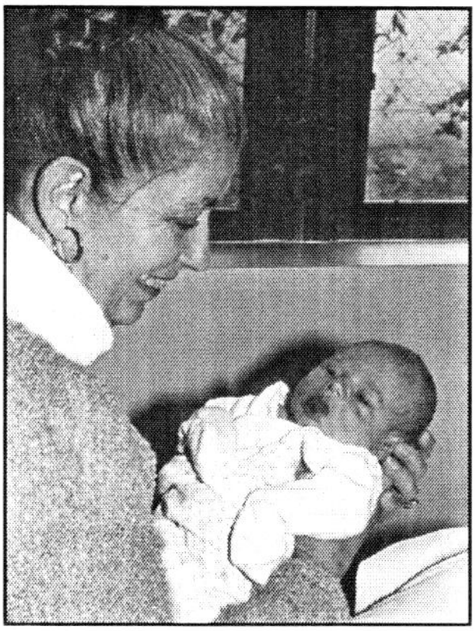

It's always been my desire to be present to deliver those patients who have come to me for care. So when I was going to be out of town for a week or two or just for a weekend, I usually had a talk with those women who were due to deliver.

"Look," I would tell them, "I'm going to be gone for the next two weeks, so let's work together on this thing and have the baby when I get back. Just tell the little gal or the little guy not to come while I'm gone because I want to be here to help bring them into the world."

Years ago Bill and I were scheduled to be in Virginia Beach for a week-long lecture session. Before I left, I told my patients, "Let's stay in a holding pattern until I get back if it's okay with you and the baby." They all agreed. The day we were ready to return home, I had a dream. In the dream, I saw all of my O.B. patients standing around me, wearing white tops and pink shorts except for one who wasn't wearing the same kind of outfit.

When I related the dream to Bill, I realized that these outfits were the O.B. uniforms that patients would be wearing in pregnancy. When a person is "in uniform," they are following orders. All of the O.B.s were apparently following orders except the one.

Sure enough, when we returned home, that is what had happened. The one woman had her baby three weeks early, and the irony of the whole situation, and yet the remarkable part of it all, was that this is one woman out of the whole group whom I had not informed about our leaving. She was not "under orders."

Dreams have had a highly important role to play in my life, and particularly in my care of obstetrical patients. Dreams can reveal the health or illness of the baby, the sex, the time when it's to be born, and much about what is to happen and the nature of the personality and abilities of the unborn child. So it has been my practice to encourage my patients to dream and report their dreams to me. The expectancy of the miracle of birth in the minds of these people heightens the psychic nature of their dream state, and the results are often spectacular.

Even the involved husband and nurses get in the act of dreaming purposefully. When I was to be out of town another time for a week, I had again instructed my patients accordingly. One of the fathers told me that he had a dream which he thought was important.

"I dreamed that I was in the service," he said. "I came up to a gate and found a little child standing on the other side of the gate. I opened the gate and said, 'Come on in.' The child answered, 'Not yet!' That was the end of the dream, but the interpretation was quite obvious.

I had other interests in the dream, however. "Did the baby tell you when he would come in?" I asked the father.

"I forgot to ask."

The dream did not recur, so the father could not ask. The baby apparently listened adequately, however, for he waited for my return from the trip.

In 1976, I was due to be gone for four weeks on a tour with Arizona businesswomen to China, and one of our nurses was due to have her baby shortly after my departure date. She took castor oil twice in an attempt to bring about an early arrival of the expected newcomer, but all to no avail. She had a dream.

"I went to sleep asking my baby to tell me whether or not he would come before Dr. Gladys left. I was in the Clinic waiting room, in the dream, and the waiting room was done in blue. In the corner was Helen Murphy and she was holding a baby. The two of them were dressed in pink. I said, 'Oh, and when did you have your baby?' She said, 'Shortly after 1:00 a.m. this morning.'" (In reality she did have a girl at just that time.)

"Then there was this baby strapped upside down (with his face looking at me) in a chair. He was in blue, and this baby was my baby. I told him to sit up straight and he replied, 'I can't sit up straight.' So I said, 'At least you can put your shoulders back,' and so he did. Then I told him to come to me and he said, 'If you want me, come and get me.'"

Her baby was born ten days after I left. It was a difficult delivery, and in a sense, her doctor did need to "go and get" the baby. It was a persistent posterior presentation, just as the baby showed up in the dream, looking right at her, and it was a boy, wrapped in the blue coverlet that the mother brought for the occasion.

Our nurses dream up a storm and they also get pregnant. Another time, one of our nurses was pregnant and under my care. She was a prolific dreamer. Up until the first or second week of November, I thought she was carrying twins because of the rate of growth of the uterus. Beyond that, it was not clear whether it was a single pregnancy or twins.

I'll try not to interpret all the symbols in the following dreams, but they seem to tell a chronological story that builds in a very interesting manner. (See if you can tell from her dreams what was happening.)

> October 25: "I was with a short fat man who had one leg – the other paralyzed, peg and cane. At Ginger's parents' old house. Walked in with man to find couple who hadn't shown up somewhere else. Weren't in kitchen. I know they were dead in living room – wouldn't go in. Sent man to look. I picked up tiny starving kitten and walked to my mom's house to call police. Fed kitten first when there, making sure to get all food from can and feeling good as I watched it eat. Then, realizing I'd better call the police asked brother Mike for phone number."
>
> November 3: "Betsy (my friend) had a dream that I had cute twin girls with red hair. Peggy and Betsy holding them . Said, 'They need blood gases.'"
>
> Week of November 12: "Earthquake – everyone holding on to furniture (in high story of down-

town building – a clinic). Betsy there, Alice, John B. Once it was over we went to lunch and everything was okay."

December 5: "Held captive by Mafia-type man (here in our townhouse). Woke up when I touched something cold – it was a skeleton. Got up and asked man (in suit) why he put it in my bed. He said there was nowhere else (no room) to put it and that I'd have to leave now feeling glad that I could leave but upset over the manner it was done. Going up to man and putting my hands on his face and saying, 'It's Faye coming back, isn't it?' (And knowing this was good because she belonged with this man.) He said a little reluctantly, 'Yes.' Was trying to hurry and collect all my things (toothbrush, combs, etc.) because it was dark and late and I knew I needed to get to sleep. Also, I knew I had to get up for team meeting and wondering how I'd get it all done and still get to sleep and be able to work. Brent downstairs playing with another man in suit. Then becoming afraid to go back to my apartment because I hadn't left any food out for my cats and it has been a month. Afraid I'd find them dead. Thinking of calling my brother Michael to come and go there with me, but knowing I couldn't."

December 13: "Husband and wife (separated) with two girls. Husband wants to take both daughters on a trip around country. One finally agrees – the other pouting, not wanting to go. I was there as an observer."

December 14: "Sitting on couch – black man came in, tall, thin, dressed very nice, colorful, black style. Sat next to me, kissed me. Very friendly, not lovers now but I knew that he had been my husband once – not in this lifetime, though. I felt love for him but more a good friendship. He had a 'white face' on and said, 'I'm going to a party – does this look all right?' I didn't care, told him to do whatever he liked, I liked him either way. Then we went flying with another couple. Nice breeze – going over river. Tree branch caught his side of plane (strange plane), looks like this:

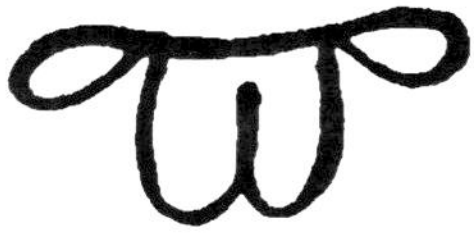

...and he fell into river washing white off face. Felt bad (all his work washed off) but still okay without it. (I had a general good feeling and happiness from the dream.)"

December 31: "Betsy's dream. Conference at Clinic – said, 'What will they do with the extra baby?"

February 10: "Judy had a baby boy on May 11 and I had a baby (boy!) on May 12. Michael and I on a large bed playing with them. Our baby rolled off edge under bed."

March 27: (1) "I had a German shepherd instead of a baby! And there was still something in my stomach."

(2) "I was in labor in some kind of O.B. office. Michael there with me. Didn't have any contractions or pain. Betsy there – delivered something (like afterbirth) and put it in pan and left. I looked down and saw two eyes and mouth in it and reached in and pulled out baby boy. Got up and walked to another room where Dr. Gladys was with lady delivering and showed her. Meanwhile Michael found another baby boy, so we had two but it was someone else's (had left it). Ended up with only one but I was confused about it all."

April 1: "Shannon, our dog, had two healthy puppies and two very small (embryo size) puppies, which died. The other two looked like German shepherds in a way.

When our nurse and I got together to bring her baby into the world, it was a boy, and there was no great difficulty. I checked carefully, for I had at one time expected twins, and so I looked carefully at the placenta. On one edge of the placenta was what remained of a fetus, very small, absorbed into the placenta tissue itself. So she did have twins, lost one of them early in pregnancy, but not really losing it, rather it stayed with her and delivered as part of the placenta.

Her dreams tell a dramatic story. She did have a boy. There had been two babies. The date of delivery was incorrect. But there are indications there about the past-life relationships with not only the one who became her son, but also the entity that fell into the river in her dream of December 14. What part do the dogs play in the dream? Well, there are many symbols in these dreams that are meaningful only to the dreamer, but she becomes the only one who can really interpret them.

Dreams sometimes are played out in our conscious life. Or perhaps it would be better to say that some of life's events are as symbolic and as meaningful as any dream could be. Another of our nurses, several years back, found that to be the case in her experience.

During her pregnancy, she remained very active and busy, working at the Clinic, until suddenly, at seven months she developed a severe case of asthma. I finally sent her home, with instructions to get some rest and told her to quit working, at least for the present. She wanted to come back to work, not only because she liked her work so much, but also because of the financial aspects of her situation.

One night she had a dream. In the dream, she saw her baby in a casket, wrapped in a plastic bag. She looked at it, was horrified, and walked away. But she couldn't really stay away. She went back, and the baby came to life, pulling off the plastic and walking towards her. With each step he grew into a handsome young man, and he kept repeating, as he came toward her, "Don't you know who I am? Don't you believe in reincarnation?" Over and over again, he kept repeating it, until she said, "I'd better start doing something!" and she awoke.

The dream was saying to her, "Look, this is saying you need to spend some time with me, your baby. You are doing all sorts of things, but you have not been meditating. You haven't spent time that you should with the spiritual part of this birth." She got with it and did the preparation that she knew was right for her and her baby.

She went into labor at dawn one morning. The hospital nurses called and told me that Cheryl was already there and in active labor. I dressed, jumped into my car, and headed for the hospital. As I was driving along Lafayette Boulevard, perhaps a bit too rapidly, I didn't see a turtledove that was resting in the road. It flew upwards, but I hit it with my car and killed it. Another dove was nearby, but I missed it.

When I arrived at the hospital, Cheryl was doing fine. I used my acupuncture needles, and the pains were eased considerably, and the labor was progressing normally. Usually, there are only three or four in the delivery room, but this time the room was crowded with nurses and student nurses, some of whom had never seen a delivery aided by the use of acupuncture.

Cheryl had already chosen the name "Jon" as the baby's name, and she and the father were both convinced it would be a boy. Then the baby was born, Cheryl took him in her arms, and without hesitation, she looked at him and announced, "His name is Jakob!"

My Biblical background gave a quick readout in my mind, and I looked around the room. Counting everyone, there were twelve present. Jakob had twelve sons. Cheryl didn't have any explanation about why suddenly her son became Jakob instead of Jon. The twelve she could not explain either. I didn't mention at that point about the turtledove.

When I arrived home later that morning, Bill and I looked up the story about turtledoves in the Bible. Obviously, my experience with the doves was speaking of a sacrifice, but what did it mean? Was there a symbolism in a life event that pertained to the birth of Cheryl's first baby? Why the name change? Well, we looked it up.

In Luke 2:22-24, there is the accounting of the story of Jesus, after he was born:

> And, when the days of their purification according to the law of Moses were fulfilled, they brought him up to Jerusalem, to present him to the Lord (as it is written in the law of the Lord, every male that

> openeth the womb shall be called holy to the Lord), and to offer a sacrifice according to that which is said in the law of the Lord, a pair of turtledoves, or two young pigeons.

The next day, when I made hospital rounds, I mentioned to her about the incident I had experienced with the turtledoves. She had to tell me the story of what had happened to her one week before that. Cheryl's closest friend called her in a panic – her father had just been taken to the hospital emergency room and had died with a heart attack. Cheryl met her at the hospital, went home with her and comforted her as best she could.

She then went to her own home, and, out in her backyard, one of her favorite places, she was just standing there, quietly, sending love and prayers to her friend's father. Suddenly, a white dove circled above her head and landed on the ground in front of her. She reached down, picked up the dove, and let it sit on her finger. It was perfectly white except for certain black markings in the corner of its eyes that looked for all the world like teardrops.

Cheryl called to Jon, her husband, asked him to come out and see what had happened, for she had never been able to pick up a bird in her hand before. He joined her, and they both talked to the dove for a while. Then they said, "You can go now," and the dove flew off. Somehow, they felt the presence of their friend's father, maybe symbolized by the dove, and they felt that they had communicated with him in some way that they could not really understand.

Well, turtledoves or not, it was only two years later that Cheryl had her second baby. Twenty-four hours postpartum, she developed a pain in her lower abdomen; eventually she was brought to surgery for an appendix that was threatening to rupture. Before surgery, however, while she was only half-awake with episodes of pain, she saw, in her extended state of awareness, a huge Monarch butterfly hovering over her like a big blanket. When it nestled down close over her abdomen the pain was relieved, and when it lifted up, the pain got worse.

The next morning, after the surgery had been performed, Cheryl was still a little sleepy. She thought she heard a tapping on the window of the room. She opened her eyes and looked and saw a beautiful Monarch butterfly floating gently in the air outside the window. It would approach the window and she heard the very slight tapping, then it would fly off. Back it would come and dance again for the new mother. After fifteen or twenty minutes, it finally left, and didn't return.

Cheryl's family lives in South Africa. Only a month after the baby was born, her father came to the U.S.A. to visit his new granddaughter. He brought me a gift – a Monarch butterfly plaque made out of semiprecious stones. Cheryl had told him nothing of her experience.

Beautiful story, isn't it? I wonder what It meant when the dove descended on Jesus' head when he was baptized. Perhaps there is more to the world around us than we are ready to admit. It is all beautiful, if we look at it with beauty.

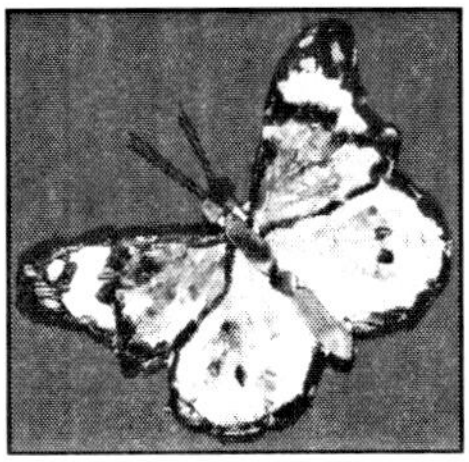

I am always impressed with stories like the following one where a baby takes control of events and is able to communicate this with their mother. The role that the father played in this pregnancy is fascinating.

> I was 35 years old, and pregnant with my first and only child. According to my OB-GYN she was due on May 13, 1990. This had been a difficult pregnancy from the beginning. I almost miscarried her one day when I was 6 weeks pregnant; it was the worst day of my life. Thankfully, she stayed. However, I had extreme nausea and vomiting the entire 9 months. We bonded very early in her pregnancy, and it was obvious to me that she was having as hard a time on the inside as I was on the outside.

One night, during the last week of January, 1990, I had the most amazing "dream." The baby called out to me in the dream. She was in a shadowy place, and I couldn't see her, only hear her. She asked me if it would be all right with me if she was born by C-Section. I told her that I was planning for her to be born through the birth canal, and asked her why she wanted to be born by C-Section. She told me that she was afraid that she would suffer brain damage if she was born in the normal way. I told her I didn't want her to have brain damage, and that she knew what things looked like on the inside of me better than I did, so if having a C-Section is what it would take for her to be born healthy and normal, that was fine with me. Then I asked her why she was asking for permission for this. She says that she knew that a C-Section would be a lot harder for me, and there would be a longer healing process and she didn't want to hurt me, so she wanted to ask my permission first. I thanked her for her consideration, and told her that I would talk to my Doctor, and tell him that I wanted a C-Section. She told me that I didn't have to do any of that because she would handle everything. I asked her how she would do that. She said that she would be born by an EMERGENCY C-SECTION. I was shocked, and asked why an emergency? What kind of emergency? She said that she wanted to choose the day and time of her birth, and for that reason she was going to be a breech emergency. I explained to her that breech births weren't considered emergencies today. She said that this one would be, but not to worry, she would be fine and I would be fine. I became a little hesitant at this point and I told her that maybe she should rethink the emergency part of this, and to consider that things may seem a lot easier to do before we incarnate, than they actually are when we get here. She assured me that she would not do anything to jeopardize her health or mine. I said, OK, and told her to tell me if there was anything else I could do to help her. I woke up immediately after the dream, and laid awake the rest of the night absorbing the magnitude of this communication. I remember feeling concerned that I might be giving birth to a control freak.

The next morning, I told my husband about what happened. He was amused and clearly didn't believe that I had actual communication with our baby that night and not just a standard metaphorical dream. So, we never talked about it again. During my next OB appointment, I asked my doctor about what a C-Section was like. (I didn't dare tell him this experience because I was one of his pharmaceutical sales reps, and this didn't fit his image of me. After my husband's reaction, I wasn't about to tell anyone else.) He answered my questions and that was that. The next appointment I asked him some more questions. He said, "Why all the questions about C-Sections? Do you want one?" I said, "No, I just think that's the way it's going to turn out." He said, "Why? I don't see any reason for it. You're doing fine except the nausea and vomiting." I said, "I know, I just think it will happen that way." Then during my first April visit, I started asking more questions about C-Sections. He said, "OK, what's really going on with all these C-Section questions? Why do you really think you're going to have a C-Section please, tell me." I hesitated then blurted out, "Because I had a dream where I talked to the baby, and she told me that she needs to be born by the C-Section or else she would have brain damage, and I said OK, and then she said that it was going to be an emergency C-Section because she was a breech." He stared at me for a few second then quietly said, "But she's not breech now. It would be hard for her to turn at this point because she's running out of room there."

I said, "Well, I don't know, but that's why I'm asking all of this." He said, "Well, OK, we'll see." On my May 1, appointment he came into the examining room and said, "Well, this is the moment of truth. If she's not breech now she won't ever be because there is no room left to turn. So, you say she's breech and I she isn't, right?" I was starting to doubt myself and said, "Well, I don't know, that's what she said." He said, "OK, here we go." He started examining me and stopped cold, looked at me and said quietly, "She's breech. But she's transverse, you know, sideways. I need for you to get an ultra sound right away so I can see exactly how she's positioned. In the next 5 days, you'll have to have a C-Section." I said, "She was right." He said, "Well wait a minute this may be a C-Section, but it's not an emergency." I said, "Yeah, well, she's not born yet." The hospital couldn't get me in for an ultra sound until 2 days later on May 3rd at 1:30. I was feeling good that morning and went to work as usual. I started feeling very strange at about 11:00 am, and called my doctor. His nurse told me to go home and rest until the ultra sound at 1:30. I did that, Then when I got up to go to the appointment, my water broke, and I immediately went into labor. I paged my husband, and he came to take me to the hospital. When we got there, my doctor came in and said, "Well, now it's an emergency C-Section." He walked over to my side of the bed, held my hand and very sincerely said, "Is there anything else I should know?" I said, "No, she'll be fine, I'll be fine, you're going to do a great job." He said, "Good, good. I was planning to." Then I watched him and my husband walk out of the room together quietly mumbling to each other.

Our daughter was born at 5:37 PM that afternoon, May 3, 1990, 7 lbs-6 oz, 19.2 inches long, with red hair and blue eyes at Scottsdale Memorial

Osborn, 10 days early. Her pediatrician, reported to me that she was the healthiest baby in the nursery.

Another interesting aside to this story is that during my pregnancy, her dad would read Shakespeare to her every night. He loves Shakespeare and wanted her to appreciate it too, so he would read various Shakespearean stories to my stomach each night. Not sharing the same appreciation for Shakespeare as he had, I would immediately fall asleep. The part about this is that the day our daughter chose for her birthday, May 3, is also William Shakespeare's birthday!!

CHAPTER NINE

Birth In The New Age

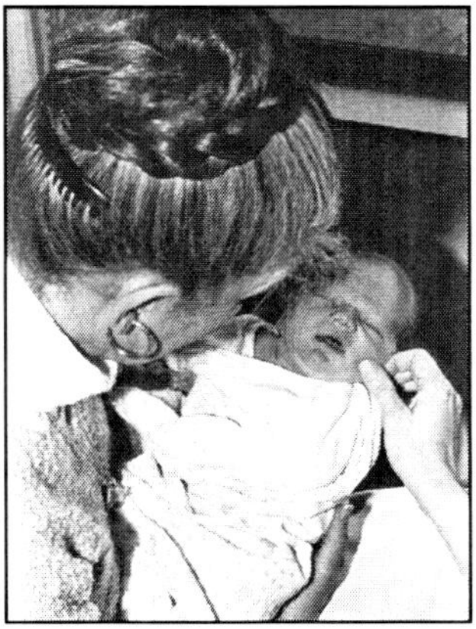

Gabriel's birth was quite an event. It wasn't the angel Gabriel arriving, but it was an important day in the lives of our whole family. Gabriel is our first grandchild.

Annie phoned me time after time when she found out she was pregnant, and each time it was the same – "Can't we have the baby at home?" Rich, her husband, was finishing up his medical school training, and the April due date made it possible for them to be in Phoenix when the baby was scheduled to arrive. So the "at home" meant the same rambling adobe homestead that Annie had lived in since she was eight years old.

My answer was always the same: "Annie, I'm just not going to deliver your first baby at home. You'll have to go to the hospital." Then Annie would feed back to me some of the things I have been saying for years about home deliveries and their intrinsic value. After all, there would be at least three doctors in attendance, Bill, Rich, and myself.

So my final answer led to our fixing up the room the way it really should be. We had a bright, sunny red carpet on the floor for our Leo daughter, green drapes for the windows. We fixed a spray of orange blossoms at the head of the bed for aroma therapy. Annie's brother, Bob, cooperated with her, corresponded with Dr. Helen Bonney and put together a tape of music to use with the contractions. The volume would go up with the onset of the contractions, down as they eased off.

We had a castor oil pack ready for use, plus my acupuncture needles, and Annie's sister Helene and her sister-in-law, Bobbie, were standing in the eaves, ready to give aid and sustenance when needed. So we were ready.

The day arrived. Annie went into labor. With each contraction of the uterus, the music built up, then eased as the contraction let up. Then, as the hours wore on, our study group members started arriving at the house, congregating in the living room. They spent most of the evening and on into the wee hours of the morning until the baby was born, visiting with each other, chatting, meditating, raiding the refrigerator, doing Yoga head stands, knowing things were going well, and just plain waiting, patiently.

The labor was a difficult one, and a long one, too. For the last nine hours, the baby's daddy didn't budge from Annie's side, supporting her back, massaging her back, putting the castor oil back on when things got tough, and giving her the kind of support she needed. "Don't you have to go to the bathroom?" I kept asking him. "No, I'm okay," was the response.

The night stretched out. There were seven people in the room, helping out, one way or another. I kept talking to Annie, helping her with the labor pains. Rich sat behind her, supporting her. Helene and Bobbie held her legs when that was needed. Bob monitored the music. Bill was supporting everything else that needed support. Finally, the moment arrived.

Gabriel poked his head out, as if to say, "Hello, world, here I am! All in one piece and ready for whatever life has to offer. Don't I know some of you people?"

Annie was crying, so was I, in between the finishing touches of delivering my grandchild. Everyone else was joining in the celebration, and Gabriel met the world.

All through the night the wind had been blowing like you wouldn't believe. In Phoenix, when we get wind storms, we really get wind storms – limbs drop off trees, all sorts of things happen. But, at the moment Gabriel took his first breath, the wind stopped.

Now I admit I have a good imagination, but everyone else noticed it too. Just ask them! The wind really stopped blowing when Gabriel took his first breath.

Bill took Gabriel while I repaired the laceration, and let the newcomer meet the rest of the members of the study group. Gabriel was introduced, and this child, this newborn baby, actually looked each one straight in the eye as he greeted each study group member. He knew, and I think he had planned, not only where he was born, but who was going to be there for his first birthday party. I think he met a lot of his old friends, from way back in time. It was a real birthday party.

We don't spank babies on the bottom anymore, and I didn't spank Gabriel. It's much more appropriate, I think, to do like I did with the first grandchild of mine – I blessed him, and welcomed him into the world. We need to be aware, as physicians, obstetricians or midwives, to be in the consciousness of blessing as each entity comes into the world.

If we do that, birth then truly becomes an exalted event, a gentle marvelous time in the lives of the mother, the father, and the infant who receives the blessing.

We need to be aware of the nature of this new being, the potential that should fill us with awe, for here we hold in our hands, as we deliver this child, a part of the Divine, fresh and new, come back into the earth to grow, to grapple with its own destiny, needing help to meet successfully the challenge of maturing into greater awareness of the Creator.

One night I was doing a home delivery for Barbara Brown who was out of town. The family was all there – both grandmothers, two of the young mother's sisters, the father and an eighteen-month-old baby girl whom I had delivered in the hospital the year before. The eighteen-month-old was asleep when we first started, but when it got towards delivery time, she woke up. Her aunt picked her up and brought her into the bedroom where the mother was having the baby and the little one was quiet and immediately intensely interested. In fact, as young children will do, they fix their eyes on a person and just stare. She fixed me with her eyes, half a frown on her face, never let her eyes move from watching me, and she didn't blink once.

I said to the mother, "I feel like the eyes of God are upon me." She continued to look at me in this intense manner until the baby was born and the father brought the baby over to her. Then she happily touched her little brother and smiled and responded.

I wish I knew what was going thru the eighteen-month-old baby's mind. I thought at first that she was watching to make sure that I did things properly, that I didn't hurt her mother or even her baby brother, but one of the therapists at the Clinic said, "Perhaps what she was doing was reliving her own birth experience," since I had delivered her, too.

It would be fun to find out what was going on in her mind. But one thing I knew, that eighteen-month-old baby was as much involved in the whole birthing process as anybody in the room. When she matures and is ready to have children, it's going to be the most natural and normal thing in the world for her to expect to have a baby without much in the way of problems. Nobody is going to be able to fill her with a lot of tales of woe about birthing because her first experience this lifetime has been one that was gentle and entirely satisfying.

We who bring babies into this world have the responsibility to become sensitive to the needs of these individuals who are under our care. I think it is important to allow each woman to have her own baby in the way she chooses. After all, choice is one of the most precious gifts to mankind from the Divine.

The method of birth, as I see it, should depend on each woman's needs as she is able to cope with her needs. Assuming there are no contraindications to what she wants, then the time has come in the world today to have the pregnant woman state how she wants to have her baby brought into this world, and we should be able to see that it happens.

It may be Mrs. Smith's method, or Mrs. Jones' method, but I suspect we will find many manners in which delivery of a baby will come about.

I like my babies born into light, not darkness. Symbolically, I think that's important. When we die, we apparently are seeking the light – if recent research with the dying patient means anything. It makes sense to me that, when we come into this world, we have gone through a period of darkness and development in the womb, and we are wanting to find that light at the end of the tunnel.

When I've delivered a baby, I see them searching for light, and when their eyes move around and find the light, they latch onto it. These are happy babies; they often smile at the world. Recently, after I'd delivered a little one and placed the baby in the mother's arms, little Angelia looked right into her mother's eyes and smiled! This baby was delivered naturally, as we call it, without medication. The mother told me that her first two children had screamed as if they were in pain during the first few hours after birth. The difference between the earlier birthing process and this one for her was, at the least, gratifying.

It may be that in the western world, we have become too deeply engrossed in techniques, and have forgotten that the quality of the delivery of a baby depends more on the attitude of the mother and those around her than on any particular technique.

Some mothers want it quiet when their babies are born, a subdued, sedate kind of a procedure. Some want music with the delivery, some want to tape the whole event. I try to cooperate with them, and encourage them.

But one special patient of mine, when she started labor, was different. Every time she had a contraction, she would grab the side of the bed and yell, at the top of her voice, "Gr-r-reat!" She was so pleased with this whole process. Between the contractions, she would be quiet.

This mother needed to express herself. She played tennis until a week before she had her baby – she was that kind of an active, involved female. If I had asked her to keep quiet because she might be bothering someone else, it would not have been right for her. She needed to yell, like a cheerleader, the "Gr-r-reat!" that let her do what she really needed to do.

Another of my mothers was just the opposite. We were not aware that anything was happening. If I had my hands on her fundus, I could tell that she was having a contraction, but not by the expression on her face. For her, this was a serious, important event that was for all the world like an American Indian having a baby in the wilds of the Southwest.

These people one really has to watch out for, because they may be ready to have their baby unexpectedly. When she threw her wig (which I didn't even know she was wearing) across the room, I shouted to the nurse, "Let's get moving!" and we took her into the delivery room. I was right, too. She was completely dilated and ready to be about the business of having this baby.

We simply cannot shape different people like this into our own likes and dislikes in the labor and delivery room and be honest with ourselves and with our patients. They are individuals and need individual attention and care. One should not expect an introvert to act like an extrovert.

The best support that I've found for the woman in labor is to ease her fears. Most women can deal with pain, but I believe – founded on many years of observation and from my own experience of having six babies – that the greatest problem is fear. I've had patients tell me, "Gee, that really hurts, but isn't this great?" Or they've said to me, "Don't ever tell me this business of having a baby is painless, but wow! Isn't it wonderful?"

Fear, however, interrupts the laboring woman's ability to cope with the pain that's involved. Perhaps the main reason we, as physicians, have used so much medication in the past is because of our own fears, and not really because of the woman's pain. Mothers can really handle that. But I think we as physicians are afraid of pain ourselves, and this fear is then projected onto the patient. Sometimes the patient is left alone and she becomes fearful of the unknown.

I have had patients who have been in labor a long time, who have had very, very hard contractions, yet who have refused medications. They just don't want it! They're moving with the contractions and understand what is happening. These patients receive the support of their husbands, the nurses, and the physician or midwife. When they have that much support around them, it makes the pain and the entire process bearable.

If the woman is afraid, if she doesn't have the support she really needs, if no one is around to help her through this time, then it may truly become the "valley of the shadow of death." She may become terrified and unable to cope with the situation, immobilized by fear.

When the husband is deeply involved with the birthing process, he loses fear he may have had, and becomes more deeply caring and supportive. He becomes one of many consciousnesses that are either giving help or creating problems for the mother in labor.

New Age birthing requires awareness of how everyone in the labor and delivery room contributes in the consciousness either a positive or negative input. The joy, the expectancy, the importance of the moment of advent into the world of a soul entering a new body helps to overcome the fears, the problems that may arise in these times

It was probably 1977 after I had done a lecture at Unity Village in Missouri that a woman came up to me and told me a most remarkable story. She said that she was in labor, December 7, 1941, (those of us who lived through this time remember vividly December 7, 1941. It was the day Pearl Harbor was invaded and we all remember where we were at that time.) She said she was having a really hard time with the delivery and the obstetrician had called in another physician, an anesthesiologist, and the room was full of nurses. She remembers that she was completely anesthetized but saw through a dimension that is hard to describe. She saw a nurse come to the door and whisper into the ear of one of the other nurses who then spoke to another nurse who then spoke to another nurse and the doctors and the other people in the room. "We're at war. The Japanese have attacked us at Pearl Harbor." What she realized in this state of animated consciousness was that each person, as they heard this announcement, shifted their consciousness and left her. One nurse thought, 'I'm going to have to go to war.' The other nurse thought, 'My son is going to be called into service.' Another one thought, 'Oh my, what is going to happen with my husband?' The doctors were struggling with the same thing as was the anesthesiologist. All of a sudden she realized that their attention and their real awareness completely left her the moment they heard this. As that happened the anesthesiologist suddenly called out, "We've lost her." She said that as she watched, immediately the consciousness of each person attending the delivery was right back in their body, right back attending to her needs, right back in that delivery room. They all worked to bring her back and she had a successful delivery. What she said to me was, "I don't know how I saw all this or knew all this but every bit of it is true. I experienced it maybe more completely than any other thing that has happened in my life and I will never forget it."

This lady's story dramatically tells us the importance of what we are thinking and doing during a delivery and how vital it is to be aware of the reality of consciousness.

Years ago, one of my patients disclosed to me that she had a dreadful fear of becoming pregnant. She had been using birth control pills for nine years. She agreed with me but did nothing when I suggested, "Mary, you know you should really stop taking these pills – you've been on them too long." So it continued.

On her next visit, I felt it was important to bring up the subject again. She finally told me why she didn't want to take my suggestion to stop the pill. "I don't want to become pregnant. I'm not afraid of the pregnancy," she explained, "and I really want children, and would enjoy having them in my home. But," she admitted, "it's not the pregnancy, I'm just scared of the delivery – real scared."

"Mary, why don't you bring some of your dreams next visit – maybe we can find out why you are afraid. It often helps." I encouraged her, and felt that she would cooperate. "We may get some understanding into the problem that has stifled your creative energy for so long."

When I mentioned dreams, she then shared with me a series of dreams that she'd had since she was a child. In the dreams, she would find herself lying flat on the ground, on her back, with her legs tied together and her arms tied tightly to her side. She was pregnant and in labor. She was alone, screaming in pain, and, in the dream, died all by herself, in excruciating pain.

This was the nightmare that had awakened her time after time since she was twelve years old. It is interesting that the Cayce material indicates that memory is stored in the endocrine glands of the body and that memories that deal with past lives and creative energy come to the awareness of an individual about the age of twelve, at the beginning of puberty.

"Mary, maybe this is no ordinary dream or nightmare. When a dream is recurrent, it means that it is important. We dream about past lives often, if we can just recognize the symbols. Maybe this is a replay of a past life when you actually were tied down and died in labor." We discussed the possibilities and some of the horrible things that have happened in the past – terrible crimes during World War II, and similar atrocities in other times, and Mary went away, thinking more about it – and with more understanding than she had had before.

Whether it was her being tied down, or a karmic situation wherein she had perpetrated such an event may never be known. She worked with a psychologist for a long time, and I saw her regularly for four years. Her real problem was the fear that's involved and the need for forgiveness of herself, perhaps, and certainly of others. About a year after this she had a normal delivery of a baby boy.

It's important, I think, to know that whatever happens, happens for the best. That the Biblical statement, "all things work together for good to those who love God and we are called according to His purpose" is a reality and deals with things that happen to people as they are seeking to do the very best they know how. This holds true in all phases of life and especially in the birthing experience. It is very easy for a young couple to fix in their minds a certain idea about how they will have their baby and if this is not followed through on, for whatever reason, they can become quite devastated.

A case in point was a young woman who had planned to have a home delivery. She went into labor five weeks early so we felt it was unwise to let her have her baby at home since we were not all that sure the baby would be mature enough to handle the home situation well. So we took her into the hospital, delivered the baby without any problem. She had the opportunity to hold the baby, to see the baby and make contact with the baby, but the baby weighed just five pounds and began to have a little bit of respiratory distress so we moved it into the nursery isolette.

Mother developed a boggy uterus and did some excessive bleeding so we started Pitocin to keep her uterus firm and stop her bleeding. I explained to her the importance of not being restricted by walls and that her love could certainly reach through the walls to the baby, and she could visualize the baby to be in her arms, cradle her, and let her know that the things that were done were done because of certain problems over which at this point she had no control, and her love was not stopped by the walls.

She went home in less than twelve hours and still was very, very unhappy about the delivery. Her statement was that her baby was taken from her and that the whole bonding process was destroyed and the whole birthing experience was a total disaster. Six weeks later, she was still hanging onto the fact that she didn't have the opportunity to have the baby with her all that time and felt that we should have broken all of the protocol and rules that are set up in cases like this for the safety of the mother and the baby and brought the baby to her or allowed her to go home at three o'clock in the morning.

It's sad, I think, that she has chosen to concentrate on what didn't happen according to her expectations and not allow herself to be involved in the joy of the birthing experience. If she had not such fixed ideas about what she expected to have and if she had not been so tied in with the actual physical bonding experience, the whole birthing experience could have been a totally fulfilling and joyful one.

Her separation from the baby was a matter of perhaps eight hours during which she and the baby were both sleeping and they could have made the contact in the realm of love that would have been every bit as profound and deep as what she could have had if she had been holding the baby in her arms in the flesh. Instead of that she still holds onto the concept that the whole experience was a disaster and no one can bridge the gap for her and for the baby. As long as this continues, the birthing experience will for her continue to be a disastrous thing.

The birthing experience, no matter what it is, can be a joy providing the mother and father allow it to be so. I have watched young women come triumphantly through tremendously traumatic experiences because they have accepted the good in the experience and not the negatives.

What of an adopted child? I have seen adoptive children who are as well rounded and loved as ones who were naturally born into a family. Perhaps the parents had to consciously work harder to bridge the gap, but with love it can be done. The child just chose another way to come into the family, and, I feel, understood – at a soul level – that he really belonged in the adoptive family and they reached their love out to him as soon as they could.

Another child found a most unusual way to be with her "mother." This is Robin's story:

> With my first pregnancy, for some reason, profoundly not fully understood to me, at about three months gestation, I miscarried. I ended up living with Mary and Michael and their two boys and baby girl. The baby girl was drawn to me. As she became mobile, I was her pal. She followed me around. In fact she did live with me at intervals and for varying

periods of time, for months to a year at one point. Once Mary stuck her on a bus and sent a letter saying she was coming cross-country! Maisy looked more like me than Mary. But we said that she was my Rent-a-kid. Surrogate mom in reverse. Then we both began using the term God-kid/God-mom (independently). On several occasions in the past I'd had the sense that this girl was the soul I'd miscarried. I shared it with Mary, who shook her head. "Yeah, sounds like something." (But how do you really know for sure?) I never told Maisy this. So, she told me in the wee hours of the a.m. when she was 16 years old, "You know Robin, I always felt like I died inside of someone before I was born."

Shudder! We then both knew…So I told her what I'd suspected and now had no doubt.

We were both awed. As was Mary.

Mary told me that she'd always known she was supposed to "give me" this kid (she had 4). Share her. Maisy had once asked her if she wanted to "get rid of her," but Mary reassured her Absolutely Not – it was just something she knew she was to do.

These parents handled the adoption in a really helpful way for all concerned and wrote me the following letter:

Before any of our three children were born, my husband and I had decided that honesty and openness about the way our family came to be, was going to be very important. We would tell them from the time they were babies that we had adopted them. Adoption would never be hidden or mysterious in our family. It would be a reason to celebrate. By the time our twin daughters were born, we had decided upon a ritual that would assure that openness.

Every birthday, as part of the celebration, we told the girls about the circumstances of our initial contact with their birth parents, the details of their births, and called it their "adoption story." We created the story that would give them the information we thought they could understand and would be interested in, based on their age and maturity as each birthday came. They came to expect the story and to know the details almost as well as we did.

By the time our son was born, we were well versed in the telling of "adoption stories," and felt that the process of the yearly retelling was as valuable to us as it was to the children. Sharing such a significant event in our lives created a feeling of closeness which we cherished. Any questions which came up were answered, and our confidence as parents grew. When our son was three, we were surprised and deeply moved by the impact the ritual had on him. His experience took us to an unexpected level of feeling, understanding, and closeness.

As I helped him to get dressed for preschool on the morning of his birthday, I began sharing the details of our initial contact with this birth mother. I told him about the call I had gotten from a lawyer in Wisconsin saying that a baby was to be born the next month. I told him about the lawyer calling the next day to tell us the baby had been born and that he was the baby. (Perhaps he had decided to be born just then because he knew his family was ready for him.) I told him that his birth mother and birth grandmother were at his birth and that everyone was very happy that he had been born. He asked if anyone else was at the hospital. I told him that since he had been born in the city which I had grown up, my parents, his grandparents, had gone to the hospital to see him and welcome him into our family. He asked again if I was there and I told him that though I knew he had been born, and very much wanted to be with him, I was in a different city and could not see him then. I told him that I thought about him, gathered as much information about him as I could, got his room ready for him, and loved him. I was anxious to move on to the joyous part of the story I knew so well. That was the part which told of the moment his father and I first met him, held him and looked into his beautiful eyes. My little boy was not ready to go on. He had something more to say. When he understood that I was not with him when he was born, he began sobbing. I took him in my arms. He looked up at me and said, "I missed you when you weren't there." In his three-year-old wisdom he knew that we were meant to be together.

Our family had come to be through the sometimes cumbersome process of a legal procedure called adoption. We all know that we are a family brought together by a much greater force.

One of the stops Bill and I made on the 1969 world tour was in England where our group met with Ronald Beasley. He talked with us for better than an hour, drawing on the blackboard with colored chalk his concept of the auras he saw when he looked at people. In most of his drawings, and he did auras for a number of our group during the session, the colors joined each other above the head in a very symmetrical fashion. But with others, there was sort of an overlapping at the top.

"Why don't the auras meet at the top in some people?" I asked.

"These are people whose souls were not tucked in properly when they were born," he answered. He expressed in words what I had instinctively known, but had been unable to put into words myself. I was really thrilled.

It means that, when a baby is born, it is our duty in officiating at such occasions to "tuck in" the aura – the way I look at that, it means simply that we have to bless that child real good! We need to handle that new arrival with gentleness and the awareness that this is a special moment in their consciousness – a transition from spirit into the material dimension. We need to be aware enough that we help in drawing the life energies, the forces of life itself, together so that the baby can adapt and function normally in this world of ours.

One procedure that has given me some trouble is the internal fetal monitor. This employs a screw which is fastened to the scalp of the infant before it is born, then connected with wires to the monitoring device. With this highly technical bit of modern scientific machinery, one can obtain a very accurate picture of the baby's condition, picking up fetal distress very early in the game, if it exists.

Such a device may save an infant's life, if a serious problem is present. But there are other ways of monitoring the fetal heartbeat and the fetal condition.

At the site where the screw is attached to the scalp, there is a point which is called the "window of heaven" by the Chinese acupuncturists, and which the Hindus call the "crown chakra." When we do not recognize energy points, then we have no compunction about going ahead with any kind of procedure, but if these are sensitive, probably very important points do exist, then we may be consciously creating harm for the child by invading territory that should be left in virgin state.

There are times, however, when it is necessary to use an internal monitor. Our daughter-in-law was not making adequate progress after a long labor and her doctor placed a monitor on the baby's scalp. Since Bobbie knew that there could be some interference with the energy pattern of the baby, she spent a great deal of time and energy explaining to the baby why it was being done, telling him that he didn't need to let it affect his pattern. From all appearances there was no ill effect. It is a reality that when the spirit is prepared, the physical does not need to be injured. She also needed some medication during the labor and was able to say to the baby, "These are being given to me and for me, not you – so you let them pass through. Don't hang on to them. We want you to be strong and healthy and you don't need these medications, but I do right now."

I once spoke at a medical meeting where a young OB-GYN physician in the room listened to what I had to say and then challenged me – "Okay, Dr. McGarey, what do you do if you have a patient that is having a problem? How do you know that you've got a baby who is in jeopardy?"

"I pay attention! I listen and spend time with the patient. As physician-priests we can use our God-given abilities and our senses to pick up distress. We can use our fingers, our ears, our eyes, and our knowingness in a way that's as accurate and definitive as a fetal monitor. And one way to this awareness is to take time to be with the mother, take time to be with the family." That wasn't all I said, but I did want to get across the idea that we are trained as clinicians, and our fingers become very sensitive in examination as we listen, as we feel, as we watch what is going on.

Each pregnancy is different. Each woman's involvement with the process is different because every woman wants to do her own thing. Years ago one of my patients was in labor and on her way to the hospital from one of the outlying areas around Phoenix.

The girl's mother called me, and she was frantic. Her other daughter, Fluffy's sister, was just killed in an automobile accident. She was herself distraught, and she was wondering, should we tell Fluffy.

"Get in touch with Milt," I told her, "and see what he thinks about it." I told her I'd go on down to the hospital and see how I could help.

Death had trailed the family closely. One of Fluffy's brothers had been killed in another automobile accident about 10 years earlier, and Fluffy and her husband had one year earlier buried their year-old son who had been born a Down's syndrome child. Now Fluffy's sister was dead.

When I arrived at the hospital I found Milt was already there, so I took him aside and asked him if he had told Fluffy about her sister. He had and apparently they had both taken the information pretty much in stride.

I talked to both of them – "I know this is a very difficult time that you're dealing with right now, and I'd like to know how you are working this out; what's going on in your hearts and minds as you are coping with this?"

"Well," she said, "I was able to release our first baby all right, and I believe in the continuity of life. I know that life goes on, and I'm trying to apply this now to my sister's accident."

The two young people there in the room in front of me were more concerned about how Fluffy's parents would be able to take the loss than they were about their own situation. Fluffy had given her sister a book about reincarnation three months before the accident. For the first time in her life, her sister, Roseanne, really dealt directly with the idea of life being a continuous event, encompassing lifetime after lifetime. She read the book thoroughly, enjoyed it a great deal, and then gave it to her parents. Her mother read the first two pages and threw it aside. "That's foolishness," was all she would say.

To help them out in their situation, I suggested that they visualize their upcoming birth as an entity changing from one dimension to another, much like Fluffy's sister was being born from one dimension to another, although we call that death. Both her sister's death and their daughter's birth were changes of dimension.

With this kind of thinking, which was helpful to them, they made it through the labor and delivery, uneventfully, releasing the sister and welcoming the daughter. Then, when the daughter was born, they both said, at the same time, "It's Molly, by golly!" And that's really her name.

A different kind of problem faced another of my mothers. She was really having a problem with her labor. It was getting nowhere. Finally, I ordered an x-ray to get pelvic measurements to find out what was holding things up.

On the way back from radiology, she asked me this question: "Where do you make the incision when you do a Caesarean?" I hadn't mentioned anything to her about a C-section.

"Why do you ask?" I queried.

"It was just a dream, but in the dream, I had been given a teddy bear for this baby, and the teddy bear had been cut open right at the bottom of its tummy. We were sewing it back up in the dream."

"You're not going to need a Caesarean," I said with a certain hollowness in my voice. "The x-rays show plenty of room in your pelvis."

She didn't make much more progress, and, in spite of the roominess of her pelvic structure, she did have a Caesarean section. Of course, the dream had properly illustrated the place where the incision had to be made. Fortunately, she had prepared herself through the dream for the operation long before I had to prepare her for it. I made a mental note to myself to stop disbelieving those crazy dreams, and pay more attention. Teddy bears simply would not deceive their owners!

One of my patients was without husband during her delivery. He was in Viet Nam, a foot soldier who left shortly after she became pregnant. She was having lots of pain in the lower back during labor, and I used a technique which I often show the fathers when they are there to help. I placed my hand on her back and said, "Now, my hand is back here. I want you to give me your pain. I'll take it. I can dump it out for you. I'm not hanging on to it. I'm not hanging on to the pain. Give me your pain now."

At this point I usually place the husband's hand there and tell him, "Now you can take it. You can take this pain for her." As they work together like this, it is a great unifying experience.

But Betty didn't have a husband there. She did bring her tape recorder, however, and I encouraged her to tape the whole thing. I kept my hand there on her back, easing it off for her, telling her, "You can get rid of this pain yourself, if you want to. You can drop it right there in the Grand Canyon. It's not far away, and it's got lots of room to take all the pain you have."

Then I told her to take a deep breath, breathe in energy, then breathe out pain. Betty worked really well with these little suggestions. She was like most women in this stage of labor. For them, the whole world does not exist. Her attention was riveted on the changes that were taking place within her own body. The contractions demanded her whole attention, body and mind. Time lost its reality for her. She had been in labor for eight hours and it seemed like a few minutes.

Her cervix was only one centimeter dilated at first. I said, "Betty, your cervix is like this," and I showed her. "It's one centimeter dilated. Let's go for one and a half. Use your mind, your imagination. See the cervix opening up. You can do it. Work at it. Feel it and see it in your mind's eye. Let yourself relax. Allow your cervix to spread so that it becomes an open cervix."

As I worked with her like this, she gradually opened her cervix, moved ahead, using her mind creatively, her whole body being in an altered state of existence and consciousness. Then she delivered a beautiful, howling baby boy. It was great, and she got every bit of it on tape.

Later on, when she came back into the office for a checkup, she told me that her husband got the tape, and there, inside a muddy tent, he and three of his buddies huddled around a little tape recorder and played that tape...and cried. It was so beautiful.

One of my families, missionaries to the Indians in Mexico, was about to be increased in numbers by one, and the time had arrived. I took the mother into the delivery room, leaving the father outside (which was necessary in those days) and the mother went ahead and delivered her baby.

Their children were all just beautiful kids, and this one was no exception. When the placenta was delivered and everything cleaned up, with the baby in mother's arms, we wheeled her cart out of the delivery room and started up the long hallway.

The father had been out in the waiting room, reading the Bible. Now he came running down the hall, Bible in hand. "Stop," he called out, "everybody stop, everybody stop. Now, listen to this –" and listen we did, after we stopped – nurse, mother, baby and I – right there in the middle of the hall. He opened his Bible to where he had "randomly" chosen a place to read while this baby was being born. It was Isaiah, the first seven verses of the 42nd chapter:

> Behold my servant, whom I uphold,
> my chosen, in whom my soul delights;
> I have put my spirit upon him,
> he will bring forth justice to the nations.
> He will not cry or lift up his voice,
> or make it heard in the street;
> A bruised reed he will not break,
> and a dimly burning wick he will not quench;
> he will faithfully bring forth justice.
> He will not fail or be discouraged
> till he has established justice in the earth;
> and the coastlands wait for his law.
> Thus says God, the Lord,
> who created the heavens and stretched them out,
> who spread forth the earth and what comes from it,
> Who gives breath to the people upon it
> and spirit to those who walk in it;
> "I am the Lord, I have called you in righteousness,
> I have taken you by the hand and kept you;
> I have given you as a covenant to the people,
> a light to the nations,

to open the eyes that are blind,
To bring about the prisoners from the dungeon,
from the prison those who sit in darkness."

We listened, and we thought, "Don't you know we are going to be watching that young man as he grows into manhood!" What a promise to be born with!

One summer, we had some Hopi Indian students at the Clinic. They wanted to spend some time observing our procedures. One girl was still in high school but was determined that she would go to medical school and become a physician.

While they were there, one of my patients went into labor, so I called the young student and she went with me down to the hospital and was there through the whole labor and delivery. It was one of those very nice deliveries – everything went well.

When it was over, I took her home in my car. It was three o'clock in the morning, and she was quiet most of the way to her home. When she got out of the car, she said, with a great deal of emotion, "Thank you for inviting me."

Suddenly it dawned on me. That's what birth really is, isn't it? It's a birthday party!

CHAPTER TEN

Planning Your Family

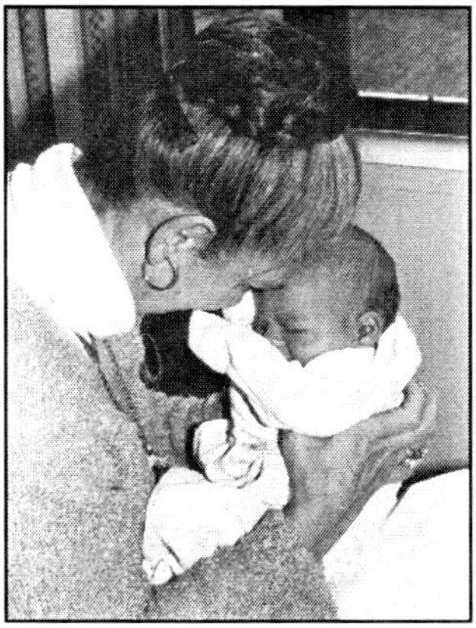

Bill and I have six children. Well, they are not exactly what you would call children at this stage of the game. Our youngest is forty, and Carl, the oldest, is fifty-three. But we have six children. It didn't just happen. Really, before we were even firmly engaged, we had both agreed that six was the magic number. From that point on, things just fell into place, so to speak.

It's what we would like to call family planning, and not exactly on an abbreviated scale.

Many years ago, I received a phone call from a student at Arizona State University. He had a group of students who wanted a female doctor to talk to them.

"I wonder if you could come down to the University next Friday night and give a talk to our family planning group?" His tone was very business-like for the average college person.

"I'd be delighted to meet with your group," I answered. "Do you think I could make it in the morning or afternoon, instead of the evening?"

"We would prefer the evening, if you could, Doctor. Are the evenings bad for you?" He was considerate.

"I'd rather spend my evenings with my family, if I could." I was trying to be diplomatic in my approach.

"Your family – do you have children?"

"Yes, we do have children."

"How many?" He was getting anxious.

"Six," I responded, as gently as I could.

Silence...dead silence.

"Hello," I finally managed, "Hello."

"Oh, - oh yes. Well, maybe some other time..." His voice trailed off. He didn't want me after all.

Perhaps, from his point of view, six children are just too many to fit into the family planning concept. However, from the facts of the case, six was correct for the planning of our family. I suppose it depends on one's outlook. It seems to me that planning the size of one's family is constructive, but the size need not be dictated from outside.

When one adds to the picture the concept of the Angel of Forgetfulness and the continuity of the individual life stream, planning gets a bit more confused, even more than the A.S.U. student thought at the time. For the entity that needs to come into a family may have more to do with it than those that plan the family think can be true. It may be family planning from the other side. It certainly must take into consideration the beliefs and habits, the circumstances of the prospective parents, the time, the place and the reasons why.

One of my patients, at my request, wrote down the following story about their experiences, which involves all of these things I've been talking about. This is in her words:

> Before the birth of Rana and Rama, I was not aware of twins within me. In the last month before their birth, I had a couple of dreams, one which I understood then, and one which did not become clear to me until later. In the first dream I saw a little girl with long hair in a playground. I was with her. In the second dream I was aware of what appeared to be an Egyptian room with a rectangular black pool in it. There were crocodiles in the pool.
>
> I gave birth of February 6, 1976, six weeks early, to twins – Rana came out about 8:06 a.m. and Rama at 8:21 a.m. He was breech. Since both children were so tiny (Rana, 1 pound and 15 ounces; Rama, 2 pounds and 14 ounces), they were rushed

to intensive care at Good Samaritan Hospital. Rana was put on 30% oxygen for the first day and then room air. Rama developed pneumothorax and was put on the respirator. Although he fought hard for his life, his lungs were not developed enough, and he passed on, on February 18, 1976. Rana, although tiny, was very healthy, and after a two month stay at the hospital, came home.

On Rama's last day of life, I gave him instructions for passage that I had read in the Tibetan Book of the Dead. I stressed that he adhere to and follow the white light. I also told him to remember Steve's and my soul pattern if he wished to return to the earth through us again, but to please allow six months to pass for breastfeeding Rana. About one half hour before his clinical death, I saw a white cloud come out of his body and I knew his soul was leaving. I felt that Steve and I had done all we could to prepare him for his passage and imprint him with our soul patterns.

That night I was at home and Steve was at a friend's house. I had a vision about eight o'clock where I saw Rama, but his body was that of a sphinx. His aspect was that of a lion and a king – he was glowing in gold and white, and he told me that all was well with him and that he would always be with me. When Steve came home later, he told me that he had also had a similar communication from Rama at approximately the same time as I.

I conceived again around August 23, 1976, just six months after Rama's death. And then I had a dream a couple of weeks ago whose meaning is not entirely clear to me, but which I will relate to you.

I was living at a school, where I had been playing a good deal of hooky instead of attending my classes. I was visiting and playing with a being of white light. The being's form was that of a small white sun which danced and hovered over

> my head. This being had the vibration of Rama. However, my sister (who lives in Boston outside of my dreams) also went to the same school and had ratted on me to the counselor. The dream ended with me entering and sitting down in the counselor's office. He and I conversed. (I don't remember the contents of the conversation.)

From her story, it seems apparent that Rama gave her just six months to prepare before he came back again, in a new and revised edition. In her dream, she was being told that she should pay more attention to her classes – the things which were there in front of her to be doing. In other words, she should take care of her body, and prepare herself so that the baby whose body was being formed within her would be well and healthy. She apparently took the advice, because he was born on schedule, weighing in at eight pounds.

At a year of age, the new Rama sits down beside his older sister, and they look like twins. It took so long for Rana to gain weight starting at little over a pound, that the two are about now equal in size.

So the mother here influenced the time when her child, Rama, should come back – a type of planning, certainly.

There was another delivery. The patient wasn't due for another three weeks, but went into early labor and while she was actively pushing, she began a kind of laughing to herself because she thought her two-year-old son was really the one that had precipitated her labor early. The way she figured that out was that he had asked for a whole list of things for his Christmas presents, and since this was just the week before Christmas and he was getting everything that he had asked for for Christmas, except his baby brother, she figured that the thing that was happening now was that little two-year-old was influencing his brother to get here before Christmas so that he would have his Christmas present. Perhaps we are much more closely linked with each other than we have thought.

The place where a child should be born seemed to be the dominant factor in this following instance, where the mother created a demand, in a sense, for a child who could accept her environmental circumstances. She had to live with the consequences. Here is her story:

> The child I wanted was a blonde, blue-eyed, slender boy who could be satisfied living in the woods and who loved his Creator. (I knew living this way could be difficult for most people).
>
> He was born in February, 1974, and fit the description! However, just before his nine month birthday the rather difficult decision was made to sell the land, move to the city, and take in foster children. (The country house was not approvable for foster care.) This decision followed dreams in which I was told there were many children in need in the city right now and there was no need to wait longer to be of service.
>
> On the night of his nine month birthday, he was sick with a high fever. I awoke as he was in a convulsion, and quickly took him to the hospital. (We were now living in the city.) At one point in the emergency room he stopped breathing. He was in convulsions for about 30 minutes. I knew I had to get down on my knees and tell Jesus Christ that I wanted God's will to be done but I really hoped my son could stay here. (The emergency people thought silent prayer on your knees and refusal to leave the room my baby was in was "hysteria.")
>
> He stayed, although he was lethargic, and his eyes were glazed and strange for many weeks afterward. He also "startled" a lot for no apparent external stimulus (this happened a couple of days before the convulsion, too).
>
> My priest and I both felt he had been facing his decision, whether or not to stay, now that circumstances had changed rather drastically from sylvan peace to a city townhouse full of lost teenagers.
>
> A few years later, when he was nearly four years old, he and I were sitting very quietly, looking

> out a big, sunny window. I had told him he was with Jesus before he was born and that he will be again, but I don't remember talking much in his presence or otherwise about his illness or my theories on it.
>
> On this particular day he had a very serious, faraway look on his face (and we hadn't talked about anything in particular). He said, "Mommy, before I was a baby, when I was with Jesus, I told him I didn't want to live in a house. So why do we live in a house?"
>
> After being "blown away" for a minute, I named some of our thirty foster children and said Jesus wanted us to help them here in the city.
>
> He accepted that, and ran off to play.

Children will often, to our relief or dismay, remember past experiences and conditions and verbally go into detail about them. Sometimes we may get a clue as to who it really is that is planning this family. We should probably be content that much of it may have been already arranged and certainly to our benefit, no matter how many or how few children we may be given to care for.

One of the many extracts from the Edgar Cayce readings dealing with the meaning of life seems to me applicable when we think about our responsibilities here or what the baby may have chosen:

> Know that life is a river or a stream which is constant, and each appearance is as a pool that may refresh, in which others may be refreshed or become stagnant and not get very far in a development in a material or earthly sojourn; or it may apply the truths of the spirit – as the ripple, as the roar of the cataract, as a part of the physical consciousness in every experience. 5392-1

CHAPTER ELEVEN

The Tree of Life

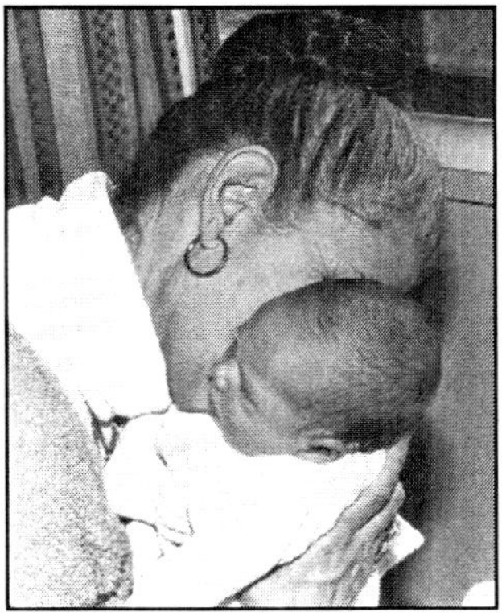

In the last twenty years there has been a great deal of research done which validates the stories which I had written in this book years ago. There are a number of books written on the subject of communicating with the unborn child. One of the beautifully sensitive books written by David Chamberlain, Ph.D., *Babies Remember Birth*, gives us insights into the process which is going on during conception and pregnancy. The following quote gives us a picture of what is happening in the uterus.

> One of the earliest hints of attentive fetal listening can be seen in intrauterine photos of a prenate, eyes sealed but looking profoundly absorbed, delicately holding the umbilical cord. This cord links the solitary womb with the surrounding world.
>
> Better than a television cable, the umbilical cord pulses with the traffic of life passing back and forth between you and your unborn. Ever-present, it is a handy plaything but alive, changing, and flooded with information. This lively conduit may be a biofeedback unit from which the baby gains information about the flow of nutrients and the slowing or speeding of circulation, a type of maternal-fetal monitor that carries reassuring or worrisome news.

I was talking to the movie actress Lindsay Wagner one day when she was pregnant with her second child. She had just come back from a class which was given by her child birth instructor for children who were expecting a new brother or sister in their family. The class was directed primarily to the siblings of the unborn child. There were charts, pictures and diagrams of the developing pregnancy both from the perspective of someone on the outside watching and that of the baby developing on the inside. Among the illustrations was a picture of the umbilical cord as it attached to the baby in utero from its origin in the placenta. When her son Dorian saw this, he said, "That looks like a tree." When Lindsay thought about this she realized that it did indeed look like a tree. Truly a universal symbol. There isn't one of us who is born into this dimension who hasn't spent close to nine months in the uterus with nothing to perceive except the walls of the uterus, their own hands, their own feet, and this amazing structure from which they receive their nourishment and a great deal of information. The structure itself is like a tree with its roots in the placenta and the limbs creating the fruits of conception in the growing body of the child. The trunk is the umbilicus.

The more I thought about it the more it seemed to me that we have a wonderful opportunity to look at this symbol, the tree of life. From ancient times it has had its roots deep in the ground and its limbs reaching up to the heavens. Its fruit grows gradually, ripens and then much like the story of pregnancy and birth, drops to the ground to start the whole cycle over again. We need to understand the continuity of life, the importance of nourishment that comes from the mother to the baby and from the divine to the child. It is interesting that God is referred to as the Father and the earth as the Mother. We are the children of this symbolic union of spirit and flesh. The tree of life then brings nourishment, both from the earth and from the heavens. The heavens give life itself to the developing child, the fruit of the union of the sperm and the ovum. From the earth, the child is nourished with oxygen, food, minerals, and chemicals. If the soil is poor, the tree does not develop well and frequently is made sick. Good soil on the other hand, creates health. Thus a baby growing in the womb with the placenta actively bringing nutrients to it, either grows in health and vigor or it becomes ill depending on the food the mother eats, the water she drinks, the air she breathes, the nourishment produced that is healthy or unhealthy. It is also the spirits in the heavens that nourish the thoughts she thinks, the movies she watches, the emotions she feels, the joy she expresses, the hope and love, faith and gentleness. All of these become part of what the baby lives and grows with. If she is angry, afraid, jealous, or working with any other negative emotions, the baby derives its nourishment from that environment and the tree of life in this manner also can be blighted.

It is exciting to me to think about the wonderful opportunity that any mother has to nourish her baby in the way that God himself nourishes us.

With our modern techniques, we now can watch what is happening as the baby develops in utero. We know that by the seventh week of pregnancy, the fetus has hands and fingers. By the fourteenth week, it can bring its hands together and may start sucking its thumb. It starts exploring, grasping, touching, and receiving information from its environment throughout the whole process.

There are signs of the ear developing within a week of conception. By the time the fetus is six months old, it has elaborate passageways and chambers in the ear with intact connections to the brain. We now believe that babies begin hearing as early as the eighteenth week of pregnancy, and by the twenty-eighth week, the baby's responses to sound are consistent. Research done in a London maternity hospital revealed that the fetus, between four and five months, was calmed by music from Vivaldi and Mozart, but was restless when Brahms, Beethoven and hard rock music were played.

In 1955, an American child language specialist, Henry Truby, was able to identify what he termed, "cryprints" which had as much individual qualities as fingerprints. He discovered that babies in the womb were hearing and learning speech from their mothers. By the time they were born they had already acquired some of their mother's personal accents and speech habits. We now know that the unborn hears the mother's sounds day and night. The sounds of her body are constantly bathing the baby with stimuli.

Paintings and statues of Madonnas almost always show the child held on the mother's left side. Perhaps this is an acknowledgment of the baby's desire and memory of the mother's heartbeat which it heard throughout the pregnancy.

A baby's nose begins to profile itself around the sixth week, is well formed by the fifteenth week and very shortly after birth can recognize smells associated with their mother.

The senses which develop and are active in utero of feeling, tasting and hearing all prepare the baby for its entrance into this world. Although the eyes develop throughout the pregnancy and are completely functional at birth, they probably do not function as sight until the baby takes its first breath. At this point though, the baby seems very anxious to recognize the people that are there at the time of its birth. I have watched babies even before the rest of its body is out, start looking around and as soon as they are able they will focus their eyes on the father, or the mother and/or whoever has been close to them and whose voice they recognize as having been present during the pregnancy.

Things that happen and are said during the delivery impact the newborn at a deep level which can be issues that the soul deals with for the rest of their life. Quoting from Dr. Chamberlain's book, *Babies Remember Birth*, he quotes Dr. Stanislav Grof who developed the conviction that labor and delivery exerted a profound, lasting effect on the personality.

> During one session, a patient reported hearing distant human voices laughing and yelling and sounds of carnival trumpets. Later his mother independently verified that this was a womb memory. She had attended the annual village fair, against the advice of her mother and grandmother. According to them, it was the noise and excitement of the fair that precipitated the delivery – a story the patient denied ever hearing and one his mother did not remember telling him.
>
> For example, a person born prematurely acts differently in the same situation than a person who was born late. Unwanted children may invite rejection, those breech-born may have trouble completing things, and incubator babies may grow up acting as if they are separated from love by a glass wall.

It is interesting to hear stories which are told about people remembering their own birth. I was talking to a man who was in his fifties a couple months ago. I had delivered him and he was telling me that he remembered his own birth. He had this vivid memory which he had experienced all his life but was never able to identify it until he was present at the birth of his first child. At that point he realized what his memory was. The memory which he had was of being in a tunnel which was very confining and he was feeling squeezed and propelled forward moving toward light and this he felt throughout his whole body. Then there came a point when he felt a sudden explosion into the light and people cheering because he was a boy.

This experience was something that he had repeatedly during his lifetime and when he told me about it I remembered very clearly because his was a family who really wanted a boy. They had three daughters and now finally the son was born and there was great excitement and cheering when he arrived. People who have experienced re-birthing or who have been hypnotized back to the time of their birth frequently describe the experience in very vivid terms.

It is interesting to me that the more we learn about what is going on during pregnancy and delivery, the more it validates what mothers have known throughout the ages.

CHAPTER TWELVE

Practical Hints – And More Stories

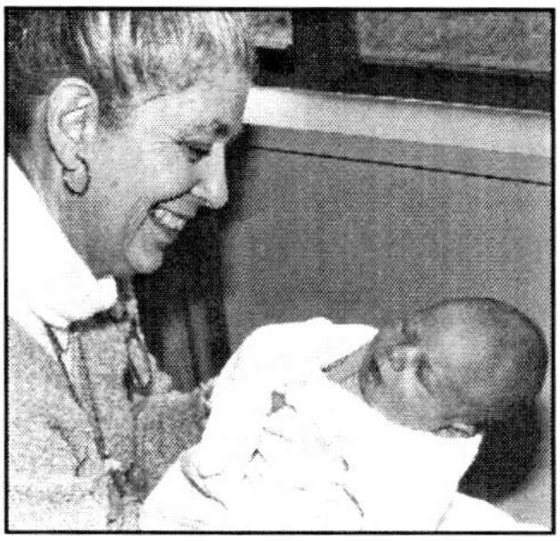

In medical school – I attended Women's Medical College in Philadelphia, Pennsylvania – I learned much about obstetrics. Some attention was paid to the ordinary things, like diet, clothing, cleanliness, exercise, and how they are important to proper care of the pregnant mother.

More attention was paid to the techniques of doing the delivery itself – and we physicians have been quite adept to this. With the advances of laboratory testing and the mechanical devices that the world of science has handed us, we are technically equipped for most any emergency.

No attention at all, however, was paid to the pregnant mother's mind, nor was it admitted that a spiritual component of the mother even existed.

In the New Age, we find ourselves with an excellent material capability to care for and deliver babies, yet there exists a marked deficiency in recognizing the whole person. This, in my opinion, leaves the medical profession of today with much to learn, if it seeks to avoid a revolution within itself.

For, no matter how skilled we may be at mechanically bringing a baby into the world, the person, in body, mind, and spirit, lies at the center of the stage. A proper delivery of the baby and proper care of the pregnant mother cannot be attended to without recognition of this whole being.

How can such a change come about? One way, certainly, is simply to recognize that the pregnant woman has intelligence, is a spiritual being, has the power and the right to choose, and can help out in this whole process of having a baby by doing little things herself that will make the pregnancy a more successful venture in the life process.

That's what this chapter is about. I'd like to tell some more stories, for human experience is where the action is, and we can learn more from the patient than we can learn from books. The patient is the ultimate source of research material – and we must always remember that we are dealing with life in its essence here, with life in its making and in its development. For there is nothing in all of creation as magnificent as conception, development, and birth of a baby.

It is important that the mother learn that her mind is creative in helping to make her body healthier, in communicating at a nonverbal level with the child she is carrying, and in helping to establish a firm, healthy basis for the growth of that baby inside her uterus.

It is important that the mother learn that the spirit can never be avoided, if she wants to be a whole person. For, as stated in the Cayce readings that I refer to so often, "The spirit is the life, the mind is the builder, and the physical is the result." The spirit is where we come from. So prayer, meditation, caring and loving one another, living the concepts of patience, understanding, forgiveness, and gentleness – all of these are food for the spirit.

In touching on some of these subjects in this chapter, I have used headings, for easier reference, and have made the assumption that whoever reads these pages will understand that I am just touching, not exploring the ideas. Hopefully, some of them may touch enough on the essence of things to be helpful in one way or another.

Castor Oil as an Aid in Pregnancy

The oil of the Racinus communis bean has been used for centuries in the care of the human being. It is known today as castor oil and its most common use in medical literature is as a cathartic. We have found a number of other uses for the oil, however, far removed from simple cathartic.

Let me tell you first the routine I used when I was faced with taking a trip and had patients who were just about due. I had the mother take some castor oil about three days before I was to leave. If nothing happened, if she didn't go into labor, then I could pretty well count on the fact that if I was not gone longer than a week, I could make it back home in plenty of time before she delivered. This doesn't always work, but it has been consistent in my experiences.

Its efficacy as therapy does not stop there, however. We use it applied to the body instead of into the body, and in a variety of ways, during prenatal care, labor, delivery and in the postpartum period.

Barbara Brown, our nurse midwife, used castor oil as a lubricant during delivery, and had the mothers rub castor oil on the perineum during the prenatal periods, to help stretch the perineal muscles.

After the baby was born, especially if there had been a lot of swelling and bruising of the perineum, we urged the mother to apply castor oil to her perineal pad. This helps in the healing process and is efficient in easing the pain and cutting down on the edema.

Using castor oil in packs is a method of therapy straight from the medical files of the Edgar Cayce readings, and I have had patients use these packs to prevent miscarriage, as a soothing application to the abdomen when they are uptight emotionally, and in ways described in a book Bill wrote a number of years ago.

One of my mothers called me one night to report that she had started bleeding. She was just six weeks along in her pregnancy, and we were both concerned. I told her to get off her feet, put the castor oil pack on her tummy, and stay in bed until the bleeding stopped. The bleeding slowed down almost immediately, and within the next two days, it stopped completely.

She got up and around in another few days, but I insisted that she keep the pack on continuously for the next two weeks while she was getting back to normal activities. The rest of the pregnancy went along normally, and her labor and delivery was also without incident. When I delivered the baby, I thought at first that everything was all right. But on looking more closely, I discovered that the baby had – not a hare lip malformation – but a healed, repaired hare lip, from the base of the nose, through the lip, the gum and into the hard palate.

The repair looked like it had been done by a master surgeon! I had never seen such a thing before, a malformation coming about in utero and being repaired while still in utero. I was excited and the nurses were excited. The mother was happy about the whole thing, but did not realize the implication of the event.

When I got home that evening, Bill and I looked up the events as they occur in the embryological development of the fetus. Sure enough, it is at six weeks that the lip is formed in the fetal life.

The malformation must have started at the same time that the events had their inception that led to the bleeding episode. The changes had to have taken place that we call the hare lip deformity. Then, when we had the mother go to bed and place the castor oil pack on her tummy, history had a turning point. The body, which can always respond to return things back toward normal, went to work and repaired the defect. What was left was a scar. You don't get a scar if there is not a defect in the first place.

It is interesting that the mother had dreams that something was wrong, and I kept telling her that everything was going to be okay. She accepted the little fellow with a lot of love, and he is growing up now with a repaired hare lip deformity that can hardly be noticed.

When I told this story to one audience, a woman came to me after the lecture with another story:

> You know, twenty-one years and nine surgeries later, my son looks like this baby looked (we had shown slides of the baby at birth), and the interesting thing is that I also spotted at six weeks of my pregnancy with him. If I had only known it, do you suppose I could have avoided all of that for my son and myself by using a castor oil pack?

Nobody can answer that question, to be sure. But it is a possibility and worth thinking about. It is not difficult to use a castor oil pack and it is rare that we ever have any adverse effects. Now and then, someone has a slight sensitivity to the oil.

But aside from the packs, the things that we do to and for ourselves physically certainly have an effect on the baby that's being carried. The food, the drugs, the attitudes – all of these make a difference in the health and the welfare of the baby that is to be born.

We've had a number of patients who have had problems with postpartum phlebitis. What I usually suggest for this condition is a castor oil pack without heat over the area involved. Usually, within 24 to 58 hours, the phlebitis is cleared up.

One postpartum patient developed phlebitis of the left leg. I instructed her to use a castor oil pack, without heat, and told her to come in the next day to be checked. When she returned, it had cleared up so completely that my associate could find no sign of the phlebitis at all. In fact, I had a difficult time convincing him that she had any problems with it to begin with.

Bonding

When I delivered a baby, I placed the infant directly into the arms of its mother. Every mother wants this to happen, so she can touch this bit of humanity she has been carrying around for nine months, hear him breathe, maybe squeal a bit, look into his eyes, hug him close to her own body, and simply feel the wonder of the moment.

This is called bonding. It is really the introduction of child to parent at the physical level, with all the psychological overtones and the spiritual reality that play a part in the process.

Early contact and closeness such as this between the mother and child might mean a big difference in the child's I.Q., as well as its ability to adapt to a changing environment, according to some researchers.

If, however, something interferes with the course of events and the bonding process does not come about, there are other ways of approaching the solution to the problem. It may not be as effective, but we just have not been able to "prove" some of these things that seem to be practical and worthwhile in human affairs. So it may be just as effective. Worth trying, in any event.

In such a circumstance, the mother might visualize the baby in her arms, visualizing her nursing the baby or feeding the baby, allowing herself to be part of the baby's awareness. In some of the magic that exists between mother and child, this communication comes about and the baby, whether in isolation or in intensive care, may understand and benefit.

Many years ago, a young lady who was about six months pregnant came to see me. She said, "Do you mind if I leave my body every so often?" I replied, "Of course, I mind. You really need to stay in your body. Your baby needs you and you have already made a contract with the incoming entity that you were going to take care of him while you're carrying him. It's important that your consciousness stay with the baby." She agreed.

About three weeks later she developed a severe kidney infection which needed medication. In spite of the medication, the infection continued longer than I had expected. One day she reported, "I figured out why I am hanging on to this kidney infection." I asked her why and she replied, "Because it gives me an excuse to leave my body." As soon as she recognized that this was what she was doing and that it was not a legitimate cop-out, she got over her kidney infection and proceeded with the pregnancy without any more astral travels or trips out of her body.

This was her second baby and when she went into labor, the baby was a breech. It was a very difficult breech delivery. Two of us physicians were working with her. As she had her baby, we had to use forceps on the after-coming head and she was completely conscious throughout the whole procedure .

Every so often she would lift her head and say to me, "I'm still in my body, Dr. Gladys, I'm still in my body." The nurses didn't know what she was talking about, but I would say, "That's great, Kathy. Hang in there," and she would go on about her business.

This experience was an interesting lesson to me. The bonding that takes place occurs not just at the moment of birth but throughout the pregnancy and afterwards, too. What this young mother was able to do was to recognize that she needed to stay in consciousness with her baby throughout pregnancy as part of the whole process.

I, myself, had my first child during those times when much medication was used in obstetrics. I was totally medicated throughout the delivery. Carl was a brow presentation and forceps delivery and I did not see him for at least 36 hours after he was born. However, this has never stopped my feeling of love for him or my joy at his presence and birth. I think bonding is a very important aspect of delivery. Its better if a mother can hold her baby immediately and not be separated from him. It's a joyful and wonderful experience.

On the other hand, it's been my experience that a kind of bonding can occur in any circumstances – like mine, for instance. We need to learn that the spirit is greater than the flesh and we are all capable of working at a higher level through any barrier that tends to separate us.

Within a 24 hour period, I had two patients who had to go through Caesarean sections for different reasons, and their stories bear repeating.

One young lady had herpes genitalis which required that she not have a vaginal birth, but rather a C-section. This is for the protection of the infant, for herpes is highly infectious.

During the time that the baby was in the hospital, the baby was never allowed to be touched by human hands directly, but always with gloves on, in an incubator, in isolation so that the infection that the child might be carrying would not spread through the nursery.

By the time the mother was ready to go home, the baby was suffering from the "failure to thrive" syndrome, which happens to babies who are not cuddled and loved, or who have other problems. The child was not eating well, was spitting up what it did eat, looked pale, was placid – it simply did not look or do well in the nursery.

The mother, though quite young in years, was wise beyond her age. She said to me, "I know why my baby's in an incubator and I know I can't touch him, but I know I can reach my love through that and I can get to him with my thoughts, and I know he's going to be okay because he understands that this is just a temporary thing. As soon as I get my hands on him, he's going to be all right."

As soon as she took him home, he started coming out of his difficulties. I saw him the next day because his mother was worried about some bumps on his bottom – thought they were herpes, and she was scared. But it was no problem, a simple skin rash. Baby, meanwhile, just a day after getting out of the hospital, was responsive, eating well, crying adequately, and his color had come back to a normal pink. He was doing all those things he was supposed to be doing.

The second mother was not expecting to have a Caesarean. But she was carrying a big, husky baby girl and there was a cephalopelvic disproportion. She just was not going to fit into the birth canal.

The surgery went well and mother and baby came out of it in good condition. The girl was a big one and vigorous. The mother had never really dealt with babies before. She was a business woman, and suddenly, she recognized that here she was in a situation where she did not know what to do. She was at a loss.

She loved her baby, but didn't know how to handle her. She nursed her for a while but didn't feel right about it. The nursing staff was a bit upset for her. "She's just not a very good mother," they said.

Here's where that old concept of reincarnation comes in again, helping one to understand the situation. Perhaps this woman was just learning how to be a mother. What if she had never been a mother before? One of the nurses said, "I'll be glad when she goes home, she acts like she owns the place. She thinks she's a queen!"

Maybe, in a past life, she was a queen. Not unlikely, for she certainly carried herself like one and she was a beautiful woman. When a queen had a baby, wasn't it a wet nurse or an attendant who took care of the baby from birth on, letting Her Majesty care for the infant only when she wanted to?

This mother, whatever her past life experiences, loved her baby. There wasn't the intimate contact that often happens, that we think is the optimum, but it was adequate. When the two of them arrived home, however, everyone in the family helped to take care of that baby, and there was no sign of a problem. Meanwhile, the new mother was learning the art of mothering in an environment that was helpful. The bonding was a different kind of a bonding process.

The Mind in Action

One of my mothers had for years been deeply involved with Eastern disciplines of meditating and diet, and these had become integral parts of her life. She was aware of different states of consciousness and, rather than take medication of various sorts during the birthing process, she altered her state of consciousness and made it through the delivery without any medicine.

After the baby was born, she suddenly started bleeding rather profusely. We packed her, made pressure on the fundus and did all the other things to get her stopped, but she continued to bleed.

"You've got to let us start an intravenous," I told her. "The bleeding is too severe, and even if you don't want medicine, you need it now." She was too weak to argue and so nodded assent.

We put a needle into one of her arm veins and started the I.V., but as soon as it started, the veins shut off. We switched to the other arm, and the same thing happened – no luck. Back into the first arm once more and meanwhile she was still bleeding heavily through her uterus. Once again the veins shut off, and I was frustrated.

Remembering all at once that Sarah had been meditating a lot, I suddenly put the whole picture together. She was unconsciously shutting off those veins because she didn't want any medicine, and she was not realizing what she was doing.

"Sarah, if you are able to close off your veins so that we can't get an intravenous started, then you can also stop the bleeding down there in your pelvis. I want you to stop it and stop it right now!"

Within 30 seconds, the uterine bleeding did stop. Just like that! I'm sure the nurses were really as surprised as I was. I didn't really think that I could have done that myself. But then, I wouldn't have been able to stop the blood flow in my veins either. So it's just a matter of consciousness, and Sarah did not have any medicine.

A friend of ours who had been in one of the early study groups in Virginia Beach when Edgar Cayce was still alive came to the Clinic years ago. She was to have a complete physical examination so needed to have some blood drawn. The nurse was able to get just a little blood when her veins shut down. She repeated it in the other veins when the patient said, "You know, Edgar Cayce said in one of my readings that I was able to control my circulation at one time in a past life and that it was possible to change the blood flow from deep to the superficial circulation. I'll try to do that now." She was quiet for a moment and the blood began to flow into the tube the nurse had already placed to receive it.

Interesting, isn't it, what we can do with our bodies? Sarah didn't need biofeedback training to manage her little act, nor did our friend from the study group. Most of us, however, would require a lot of instruction on the unconscious level, working to learn how to control involuntary functions with our conscious, voluntary mind. But things like this are a part of the New Age – capabilities of communication with our unconscious selves and with others in ways that are not very familiar. It is really part of the heritage of every human being.

Another patient of mine understood the concept of working with and contacting the baby and the activity that was going on within her uterus. She came to me when she was seven and a half months pregnant because she had begun spotting and the gynecologist, on doing an ultrasound found that the placenta was right down at the mouth of the uterus and was almost completely covering the cervix. When the cervix began to thin and began to stretch the placenta, she began to bleed. The gynecologist had sent her home to bed hoping that the baby could stay in the uterus at least a week or two longer. I suggested that she use a castor oil pack over her lower abdomen without any heat and while she was doing this visualize the placenta moving up and away from the cervix. She was very good at visualizing and understood what I was saying. She went home, put the castor oil pack on her abdomen and stayed down for the next week. Fortunately, she had help at home and was able to do this. Repeatedly each day she talked to the placenta and asked it to move. The bleeding stopped. When she went back in for another ultrasound, the placenta had moved almost completely off the cervix and the cervix had begun to thin normally. She carried the baby to term and delivered a beautiful red headed nine pound baby boy.

In pregnancy, a mother can learn to become aware of the baby's heartbeat as early as four months into pregnancy. In our prenatal classes, she learned to relax and then contract certain muscle structures in preparation for birth. Some of these muscles are not normally under conscious control. Pain can be successfully alleviated through conscious control of the pain message to the brain. Use of methods like these help the mother who is in labor and having her baby.

The mind came into action in still another manner with Gloria. Her father had died when she was 18 years old, but she still missed him, for she loved him a great deal. During the early stages of labor, she began to cry. Her husband wanted to know what was wrong.

"I'm all right," she said, repeating it again. Then she said, in a low voice, "I'm seeing my daddy."

Gloria, in that strange state of consciousness which often happens early in labor, was apparently making contact with her father who was telling her (as she told us later) that everything was going to be all right.

At the time, we did not know that she was going to have any problems. She sailed through the labor without incident, and had her baby. But then, in the postpartum periods, she started flooding – and she had to be taken to surgery to get it stopped.

Perhaps it was important for her that her father communicated and told her of the upcoming problem and that she would come through okay. This kind of comforting, assuring love and communication undoubtedly helped her to sail through the next few days, because they really were tough. She feels that she is a stronger and more compassionate person, now, as a result of the beautiful experience arising out of the pain and suffering of those three days.

Sometimes, we tend to think that if we are really doing the "right" thing, living the life that we should, that life is going to be smooth. That's really not the way things are. None of the wisdom from our religious heritage says that's the case. We need to learn in this life of ours, that life becomes the opportunity for us to gain those experiences that let us learn, and when we gain that knowledge, once applied, makes us better people.

The unconscious mind is always awake and active, and communication from parent to infant at the unspoken, unconscious level, always has to be considered as being possible. Emotions seem to be so easily transmitted, too, to bring about changes in the physical body.

Some years ago, I delivered a baby for a mother whose husband was having a lot of problems. Despite everything we could do, the child died three days later. A post-mortem showed that there were seven peptic ulcers in that infant's stomach and this was the cause of death.

Throughout the pregnancy, the mother was disturbed and upset and under a great deal of stress because of her husband's financial condition. His problems soon became insurmountable, leading him to psychiatric care and eventually hospitalization.

The parents learned from experience – they learned the hard way, certainly. Perhaps the child, having such a short incarnation, also went through a soul learning experience. The law of cause and effect seems always to be around for us to use, and it dictates that we experience what we have created. One of the Cayce readings points toward that concept:

> For, remember, it is not all of life just to live nor yet all of death to die. For it is self that one has to meet. And what ye sow – mentally, spiritually, physically – that ye will eventually reap. 257-249

In one very real sense, we can say that we always have the potential of meeting ourselves, even though we may just be a newborn babe.

An example of this is the following letter which our daughter-in-law wrote while she was in labor.

> Well, whether this sweet baby makes his/her arrival today or whenever, I have learned a very valuable lesson. This baby – although seemingly so very much, "mine" and part of me, is not mine – but rather a child of God. What I mean may sound obvious to you but being pregnant brings a time of introspection to me like no other – for I am merely me – I am forcefully made to feel (allowed to feel) part of the creative universe – part of the God-force always at work. This baby who has grown within me and shared my body, my food, my oxygen, my breath – this baby even now is independent – for I have no control over it. I cannot choose, for example, when I precisely I want it to be born – a lesson for our whole lives together – I cannot choose its life path. Oh certainly, I can guide and suggest and direct, but I can't protect from sorrow or estimate what will actually happen in life. I must now – before it is born – accept her/him as God's child (as a child of God) and give the "control" to God. My faith is stretched in this situation like never before. I hang on a cord of trust which is God as my baby lives on a cord of life within me.

I remember a poem I wrote a long time ago (eight years).

And so to children's souls around me
This is my song I sing for you.
Some day as part of my loving
My man and I will call for you.

Some day my man and I will want you
Some day together we will find
That the children who have been waiting
Have come to share our joys in time.

Together we can bridge the chasm
Together all our love we'll share
You and I and God living
We'll come together and learn to care.

We will find such laughter waiting
And I'm sure we'll find some sorrow too
But as our journey keeps on moving
All our dreams we'll give to you.

And when we come to different highways
And when we go our separate ways
We will have left you loving children
Love and strength for all your days.

And so to children's souls around me
Come and sing this song with me
Sing of happiness and loving
And know you always will be free.

Bobbie G. McGarey

CHAPTER THIRTEEN

Special Children

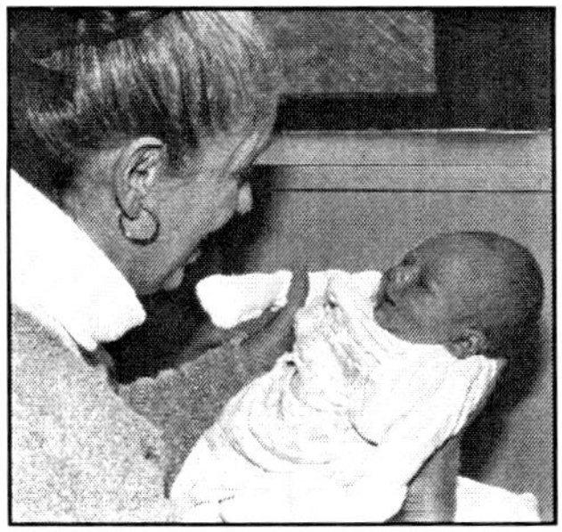

A young osteopath and his wife, who was physically, emotionally and spiritually a very strong person, wanted a special child. For years they had been studying the Cayce material, and Bill and I had watched while they prepared themselves for having a baby.

They exercised, they ate a good diet, they took treatments themselves to keep in good shape, they meditated and they kept their minds active in a constructive attitude, as much as they knew how. They prayed for a "special" child.

Pregnancy became a reality, and they continued with the positive approach toward health of the physical, mental and spiritual. Then came the big day, and Tara was born. It was a normal pregnancy and normal delivery, but the child was not normal. She had multiple birth defects and they were very serious.

Tara's mother reacted. "This kind of thing happens to somebody else, not us," she told me in a letter. "Although we knew something wasn't right, it took nine months before we got the diagnosis confirmed that Tara had a rare chromosome disorder with a serious heart condition, that only three others were ever known to have. (None of them lived to be more than a year old.)"

She continued, "I felt so torn inside, guilty too, because I loved her so right from the start, yet I had a real difficult time accepting the fact that she had chosen an imperfect body. I blamed myself at first thinking it was something I did or didn't do during my pregnancy, but woke up to realize Tara's message to us was, "Hey, this has been my choice, you know. You have no reason to feel guilty."

Right after the baby was born, the father was deeply upset, too, and went home to get some rest. He fell deeply asleep, and had a dream. In the dream, there was a scrawny, mangy-looking little tiger kitten with a cast on one leg. The tiger kitten was going around from one couple to the next, asking to be taken in. None of the different couples wanted her. No one wanted the responsibility to care for this animal. Then the tiger kitten came to Darryl and Kathy and they both said, "We'll take care of you. We want you, even if these other people don't." In the dream they cared for her and fed her and loved her very much and she grew up to be a graceful, sleek, beautiful tiger, all because of their love. Although they knew they could not contain her nor really control her, they knew that she returned their love.

Toward the last of the dream, it became obvious to Darryl that those who had refused to care for the tiger kitten now envied them.

When the new father went back to the hospital, he found that the pediatricians had taken the newborn baby and, because of the problem with her hip, had put a cast on one leg, just like the tiger kitten. Then it was that they knew they really had a tiger in their family, but they would love it and things would turn out right.

The two parents did much in the way of physical care for their new child. They followed many suggestions in the Edgar Cayce physical readings that would be appropriate for a condition like this, and these things along with the love they showered on the baby, undoubtedly accounted for Tara's living to be 2-1/2 years old before she died.

Long before Tara died, her mother had a dream about being in a rectory with Tara. The dream in her own words:

> When Tara was 16 months old, I dreamed that the three of us were living in a rectory (but it seemed it was also our lake home) when a fire broke out. I panicked and ran for the door when I remembered – Tara. Charging into her room, I grabbed her from her crib and lovingly and carefully wrapped her in our big green blanket. Then I proceeded to kick out the window and we made it out safely.

Kathy continued her story.

> When Tara was 2-1/2, she died. That night, when I found her with such a high fever, I picked her up and ran around until I found that same green blanket to wrap her in as I took her to the hospital. The same blanket that I dreamed about.
>
> On the morning of January 2nd, I had this dream: I had parked my car in a big parking ramp to go shopping. Upon parking it, I changed my mind and wanted my car back NOW. I looked at the ticket to check the location of the car and it said: Tara Christine. When I asked the attendant if I could get my car now, she shook her head and said that she couldn't release the car for two hours. I turned away disappointed but thought, "Well, I'll just go home and wait."
>
> Tara died that day. I feel that this dream was telling us that yes, Tara would most certainly be released (healed) but that we'd have to wait. The car (meaning her physical body) would not necessarily be the vehicle Tara would choose for her healing to come about. Again, we must be patient and trust.

Although Darryl and Kathy felt that the entity would not be healed in that body, it is my opinion as I read their dreams that this individual was indeed a "special" child, an entity that had a very heavy load to carry into this life. The tiger, the fire – both tell of adrenal energies that had been misused.

But the beautiful part of the whole story is that both the parents were willing to take on such a task of love, to accept a "special" challenge, to assist an individual (whom no one else would take in) to enter this life and put at rest many of the problems that had been created in past lives. It was that overflowing love that did it.

Kathy had more to say about the event, for she wrote me several long letters. "Death has a very positive side," she wrote.

> …the way it brings out the highest self in all of us and jars us into examining relationships with

self and loved ones, along with questions as to life's purposes. Tara knew that this heightened awareness could best be accomplished by the impact her death would bring, and a greater impact was felt by her leaving as a child.

Another good thing that has come about is my opportunity to share these meaningful thoughts and feelings. It helps very much to get my thoughts down in writing in order to sort out all of my feelings at this time. I could be compared to a bottle of soda that has been shaken and opened. I've kept a lot inside and now I'm ready to share. It's our opportunity to help others deal with their lives with a more positive and meaningful approach.

I never thought I'd be able to handle death the way in which we have. I guess it's proof that the laws do work, that what you generate returns to you. When sadness starts to creep in, we replace it with thoughts that Tara is no longer limited by her physical body and we don't wish her to regress. We are lonesome for her, and that's okay too, for we must learn to accept and experience the physical part – for that's where we're all at now. But our prevalent feelings are peace, joy, happiness for the three of us, and love that knows no time or space.

My one message to parents of all children, any kind of children, is a beautiful work, *The Prophet*, written by Kahlil Gibran, which reads:

"...speak to us of children. And he said: Your children are not your children. They are the sons and daughters of life's longing for itself.

They come through you but not from you. And, though they are with you yet they belong not to you.

You may give them your love but not your thoughts. For they have their own thoughts.

> You may house their bodies but not their souls, for their souls dwell in the house of tomorrow, which you cannot visit, not even in your dreams.
>
> You may strive to be like them, but seek not to make them like you.
>
> For life goes not backward nor tarries with yesterday..."

Darryl and Kathy housed Tara's body for awhile, certainly. It was not easy, for in addition to the physical handicaps, her emotional state was tumultuous. She was often a very angry child who would not allow anyone else to handle her except her parents. It wasn't until her second Christmas that Tara began to relate well with her grandparents. Until then, Tara would not allow even a babysitter to care for her.

So the tiger-kitten found a home, and someone to love her, so she could overcome many things. Isn't that what life is all about?

Last year, 1999, at Christmas time I was mailing some packages and standing in line at the post office. A woman came up behind me and kept looking around and finally looked straight into my face and said, "Are you Gladys McGarey?" Then she said, "I am Tara's mother." Immediately I recognized her. She had been driving through Scottsdale on her way to California. She wanted to mail something before she got to California so she had stopped at this post office at this time to mail her package and was in line behind me. I was surprised and delighted to see her, and she said that she had needed to follow up on Tara's story. She told me what had happened in the meantime and I asked her to write it up for me. What she wrote follows:

> Two years after Tara's passing I attended a healing service. I wrote Tara's name on a card and placed it in the box designated for those who had 'crossed-over.' After the service, the woman who got Tara's card asked me if I was Tara's mother. She then told me that when she started sending healing to Tara, she heard the words, "I don't need this

healing, please send it to my mom." Even though I found the story interesting, I didn't quite understand because I always thought that *my* job was to heal my daughter, physically.

Three years later I was attending a spiritual conference in Southern California. While walking in the desert one afternoon during silence and fasting the words came – so easily and humorously. "You've had it all turned around. *She* came to heal *you*. She was fine, not perfect, but okay just the way she was. And, *that* is her lesson to you."

Only then did I comprehend the significance of the healing service incident. With a smile in my heart I returned to my seminar and shared my wonderful break through. Mission accomplished.

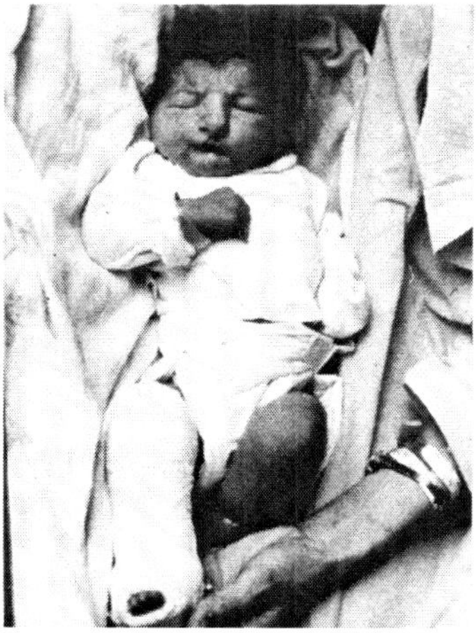

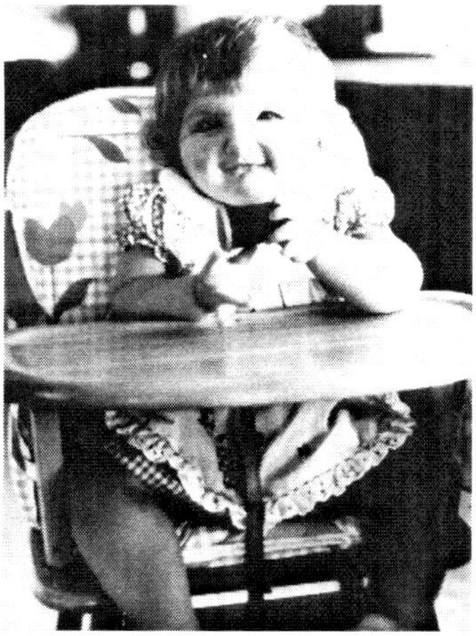

The Golden Lady

There are not only special children, but also special situations. The following story came from a woman who found this situation when she was working on her master's degree in Special Education at Cal State. She took one course that covered various handicaps in children and the effect these had on the parents in the family.

A group of parents came to talk to the members of the class – men and women who were parents to children who were classified there as "vegetables." One of the women there told my friend about her son, who was at the time seven years old. The mother was happily looking forward to the birth of her second child.

When I heard the story, I thought of Tara and of Jackie Johnson, whose story follows this, and of the many children I've seen where love and care, touching and working with the physical body and with the mind and soul has brought about wonderful changes in the lives of many people.

> They showed us a picture of the boy. He wears special (steel) leg braces fastened under his arms. I would guess he shuffles rather than walks, but is ambulatory. He wears a football helmet to hold his head upright, but owns a handsome smiling face.
>
> When the boy was born, the doctors told the young parents that the child would be nothing more than a vegetable his whole life. They consulted other doctors only to get the same opinions. The parents were advised to institutionalize the child and forget about him.
>
> The mother, at this meeting, stated that she refused to accept these opinions and for the next 18 months did everything possible to teach the child to simply hold his own bottle.
>
> Not only did she have to admit defeat on this goal at the end of this time, but her marriage was on the rocks. Also, because of medical expenses, the couple was $12,000 in debt. There seemed to be no way out.
>
> The young mother had absolutely decided to first kill the child, then herself, after her husband left for work in the morning.

> That night, when she went to bed, although she did not consider herself religious, she cried to God, "How could you do this to me?"
>
> "That night," the woman said, "a beautiful radiant, golden lady appeared at the end of my bed. The angel, if that's what she was, said, 'This was not done to you, it was done for you.'"
>
> The mother stated that she awoke in absolute peace. She felt happy, tranquil. She began to see her baby differently. Noticed that he was happy. He always smiled even when the doctors who had caused him so much pain came near.
>
> I would assume other things in her life improved. She told us her own mother later reminded her of a dream she had long before she had any idea of the facilities and aids available to these children. The dream was of the child going off to school, in a yellow checked shirt, being picked up by a school bus with some steel crutch-brace affair which fastened under his arms.
>
> This was the exact picture that became real years later as he left for school and the school bus picked him up.
>
> She also tells us that although he has a 5 to 10 word vocabulary, his teacher once told the mother that for one hour he was absolutely verbal and lucid, talking about happenings at home. The teacher was not even going to tell the mother, thinking he had these lucid periods before. The mother has never witnessed this but is in hopes it will repeat.

A wonderful story, isn't it? Sometimes, in the darkest moments, that Golden Lady makes her appearance, and the picture of life takes on new colors and new meanings.

Jackie Johnson

Jackie was born deformed. His mother was a young, unmarried girl who did not want to be pregnant, and certainly did not want the responsibility of taking care of a child. Jackie was destined for the Children's Colony in southern Arizona, where those "vegetable" children are placed.

Jackie's head had not developed properly. He had what we call hemihydrocephalus – the left side of his head was almost twice the size of the right side. His face was expressionless when we saw him first at ten months of age; he was almost totally flaccid, could not sit up, lift his head up, or even turn over.

He was unable to see, apparently could not hear, was unresponsive to stimuli of all kinds, and managed to continue living because he was able to swallow when he was fed, and his kidneys and bowels would function.

There was not room in the Children's Colony when Jackie was born, so the state placed him in a foster home, under the care of people who were members of the A.R.E. and who just did not believe that there was nothing that could be done for Jackie. They knew that every human being is going through a soul experience no matter where he is or what sort of a body he was born in.

So, Jackie ended up at the Clinic and his foster parents wanted to know, "Isn't there something we can do for this child?" Jackie didn't look much like one who could gain anything, but there was no destiny for this little fellow except the Children's Colony for the rest of his life, and Bill and I both felt that we should institute some kind of creative therapy program while he was waiting to be placed.

Bill looked up the information in the Cayce readings about hydrocephalus. It talked about energies leaking out from the bottom of the spinal cord – "nothing like this was ever taught to us in medical school," was Bill's remark. But then, when we checked Jackie more closely, we found he had a spina bifida occulta, which is an improper closing of the lower part of the spine during embryological development, which sometimes will leave the spinal cord exposed at birth with very little protection. Jackie's spine was not that severe a malformation, but there was the defect in the bony structure.

In the Cayce information, there was a suggestion that massage alongside the spine on both sides was one therapy which would be helpful for this child. Cayce did not see hydrocephalus as untreatable, and he never suggested in his readings that any kind of surgery should be done. His concept of therapy was to restore the physiological functions back to normal and these would then restore the normal growth patterns of the body.

So we instructed the foster family in proper massage of Jackie's back, as it was suggested in the readings given by Mr. Cayce many years ago. They were to start at the base of the skull and massage alongside the spine down to the level of the 9th dorsal vertebra; then massage from the coccyx area alongside the spine up to the 9th dorsal. During the massage, I strongly suggested that whoever was doing the massage keep a positive attitude throughout, and either that person or another should read something spiritually uplifting, repeat an affirmation, read from the Bible or do something that would keep the minds of those involved in the therapy directed toward the relationship between Jackie and God.

We also instructed them in the use of castor oil packs, in how to prepare for him the best kind of diet, and most of all just waited as they simply loved that little boy. Our entire staff became involved in Jackie's care, for the receptionists, the nurses, all contacted him and his foster parents, and exercised their own kind of loving therapy on Jackie.

Jackie got started on all of this kind of treatment during his first visit. He returned a month later. I was examining him when I suddenly realized that he was following my silver watch band with his eyes. Jackie could actually see! Not much yet, but he could make out bright objects and would follow them with his eyes and his head.

By the time he came in for the next visit, he was holding his own bottle, and changes continued to come about. As he responded to the treatment, he gradually came to be able to hear, he first sat up, then stood, and tried to walk. As Jackie grew, he seemed to become more and more normal. His head abnormality gradually lessened until it was difficult to tell that there was actually a hydrocephalus there.

When he was a year old, and just showing the first of these dramatic changes, we presented him at the medical symposium which we sponsored every year. Dr. Ernie Pecci, a psychiatrist from northern California, was present at the meeting. When he saw what had happened with Jackie, he was really excited. When he returned to his home duties, Dr. Pecci instituted some of the methods used on Jackie, and has found the results to be satisfactory, and so life changing, that it has provided him with a continuing research effort to establish more information about why this change should come about.

By the time Jackie was four years old, he was a smiling, happy child, trying really hard to walk, having been fitted with orthopedic shoes by another doctor who was interested in his development. His foster mother was very creative with Jackie, and I thought you'd like to read the Christmas letters that she helped Jackie write – she's told us we could do this.

To Doktor Gladiz, Dokter Bel, and Everbudy
When I wuz just a little boy, I wasnt very nosey,
I had so many problems that my future wuznt rosy.
And on my one-year birthday, I really wuz a square,
I couldn't see right, sit or stand – and didunt evun care.

And then, will yu believe it, out of all the Toms and Harrys
I was allowed to be the one to GROW with the McGareys!
Theyve got me having back rubs, up and down my spine,
Guess "massage" is whut they call it, and it really helps
me fine.

In 3 weeks I wuz sitting, by 4 weeks trying to crawl –
I also learned to stand up – holding on, or I wud fall.
And then one noon at lunch time, Momma scared me by
yelling "Jack,"
Cause for the verry first time I had looked directly BACK!!

Now I see things and I do things – I bounce and sit and
stand –
I'm evun walking pritty good with just a helping hand.
I like to visit Doctur Bel and Gladiz, cuz yu see –
Their office is just filled with LUV, Oh lucky lucky ME!

I sure like nursey Pat – but Mom sez Pat's "hard as nails,"
Cause when Patty wants to weigh ME – Mom haz to hold
Me on the scales.
And even when Pat's buzy, I still cant seem to win,
Cause nursey Arlene makes me STRIP, and weighs me in
my SKIN!

Theyve got a new recepshunist, Ive only seen hur twice,
I all ready like hur very much because she is so nice.
Jim McCready is the manager – he MUST manage a lot –
But the only thing I've seen him dew, is MAN the coffee
pot!

Oh, youre SOOO pretty Docter "G"
When I grow up, please marry me!
And Doctur Bel, I love yu too,
In my NEXT life, I'll marry yu!

****

I LUV yu ALL – I hope you KNOW
So MERRY CHRISTMAS,
Luv,
Jackie Joe (December 25, 1969)

MERRY CHRISTMAS
from
Jackie Johnson, Esq.

My friends and I've had a busy year, as all of you must
know.
I have so many things to do, I'm ALWAYS on the go.

I start the morning early, with a bottle – milk, not booze!
Then after it's all finished, I turn over for a snooze.

When I wake my folks up later, I get a laugh or two,
Mom looks like Ebenezer Scrooge – My Dad, Mr. McGoo.

Morning is my quiet time, I don't cause much alarm,
By the time lunch rolls around I turn on all my charm.

Mealtime is the best of all, cause everyone is there.
I kiss, shake hands and patty cake, and "throw it in the air."

In afternoon it's nap time, but I just CAN NOT see,
If Mama is SO TIRED why she gives the nap to ME!

It always seems that suppertime comes soon after my rest,
And then it's time to watch TV – I like commercials BEST!

Some TV shows are pretty dull, and some make lots of noise,
So when I tire of watching it – I go hunt for my toys.

I put them under the playpen pad, so that's where I usually peak,
I have to keep them carefully hid, cause the DOG likes the ones that SQUEAK! !

Sometimes I get real noisy when they're all watching TV
Of course the reason simply is – I'd rather they watch me.

My Dad looks like a grown-up, but it isn't time at all.
He's always making me sit down to roll or throw the ball.

And when it comes to bedtime, I admit to a FEW faults,
If I'm not really sleepy, I just practice somersaults!

To be a spoiled little boy – from MY mind could not be FURDER,
But visiting GRANNY and Bob-Bob, I get away with MURDER!!

I've got two great big SISTERS – but yuky, yick and blat!
They kiss me, and they hug me, and AWFUL things like that ! !

I LOVE to see "Gladys," she's usually lots of fun,
But when I need a shot – BRUUTHER – you should see her RUN!

And DOCTOR BILL's no better – in fact, he's even worse,
He teleports right from the room, and sends in some poor NURSE!

I'm "unengaged" to PATTY and I'm saving ALL my dimes,
I'd like to marry her some day – she sure does "RING MY CHIMES!"

Although I'm "unengaged" to PAT – I look around, it's true,
And of the places I like to look BEST – is at MY Receptionist SUE!

I'm attracted to Nurse Jackie, but if it's all the same –
I'd rather NOT go out with a girl who doesn't have a GIRL name!

The Ladies at the office are pretty as can be,
I don't know what all of their names are – but they sure are nice to me!

Well – LOVE and KISSES, and all that MUSH.
Me and MY FAMILY wish you a MERY CHRISTMAS.
(December 25, 1970)

About the time he was four, he was placed in the Bedell School for Special Children, and he continued his slow development, with occasional episodes of illness that brought him in to see us.

Early one morning, when he was past five years of age, I received a phone call from Mrs. Bedell.

"Jackie has a temperature of 105."

Well, Jackie had temperature elevations before, so this was not that unusual. I told her to sponge him down and give him a little aspirin, "and let's see if we can't get his temperature down."

Fifteen minutes later, I received another phone call from Mrs. Bedell – "Jackie's dead."

Bill and I did the funeral service for Jackie. This was a really important person in our lives, too. We used the story of Jonathan Livingston Seagull – it seemed to fit in with Jackie's story. Here was a soul who had come in with a special mission. Maybe we can't identify the mission 100 percent, but here he was, present with us for a short period of time. In that time, he did a tremendous amount of good for the world. The work he inspired in northern California continues to this day, and we don't know how far the impact Jackie left on the world will go.

When he first came into the office, Jackie was very ugly. He would come in and people – you know how they are – would look at him, then would look away. Then they would look back again. They couldn't stand to look at him, yet they couldn't stand not to.

He gradually improved so much that he became the darling of the whole Clinic. Everybody loved him; he'd come into the office and people would play with him. He made his transition on that note. He was adored by many people.

We let Jackie go, along with Jonathan, and we marveled that one person, in such a disturbed body, could make such an impact. We thought, "That's the end of Jackie's story."

But, no. Last year, one of the sisters who had worked so closely with Jackie came into my office. She was pregnant, and, since she was not married, she decided that she was going to have an abortion done. We went through the process of making the arrangements, and she arrived at the doctor's office when the surgery was to be done. Sitting there in his waiting room, however, she just couldn't stand the thought of losing her baby, and she said, "I just can't do it!" And she left.

This pregnancy was pretty normal until the last trimester. Then she had many problems requiring bed rest and castor oil packs. During her ninth month, she came into the office and told me this dream: "Jackie was standing beside me in the dream, and I said to him 'What are you doing here?' He said, 'I'm here!'" That was the dream.

"Isn't that interesting," I thought. "I wonder if this really is Jackie that is ready to come into this family – he's been gone now for six years." Then, I forgot about it – too wild an idea.

The child was born – it was a girl. No problems that I could tell, and mother and daughter Ann went home from the hospital in good spirits. When they came in at one month for the baby's check-up, however, I noticed in irregularity in her back – at the level of the 12th dorsal and 1st lumbar vertebra, there was a slight angulation that created a little hump there in the middle of her back.

"Your baby's fine, except for this little thing in her back," I told the mother. "I think you should start working with her back at this point and get things back to normal. Why don't you massage her back, starting at the base of the skull and massage down to the shoulder blades; then start down at the coccyx and massage up to the shoulder blades, always using a positive affirmation with the massage."

"Like I did with Jackie?" she wanted to know.

I had forgotten. It was the same, wasn't it? Was this Jackie coming back to take up where he left off? I wondered and I watched.

One of Ann's babysitters wrote me a note about this little girl whom she was very interested in, probably for the same reason we were.

> I started watching her at two weeks of age. Her legs were very rigid. She screamed when I would change her diaper and bend her legs up. Until the last two weeks, she would not use her legs at all. She still refuses to sit up. I've sat her in high chairs, walkers, baby swings, and so on. She just screams bloody murder. To me, she acts as if she is in pain or cannot control her legs from her hips down.

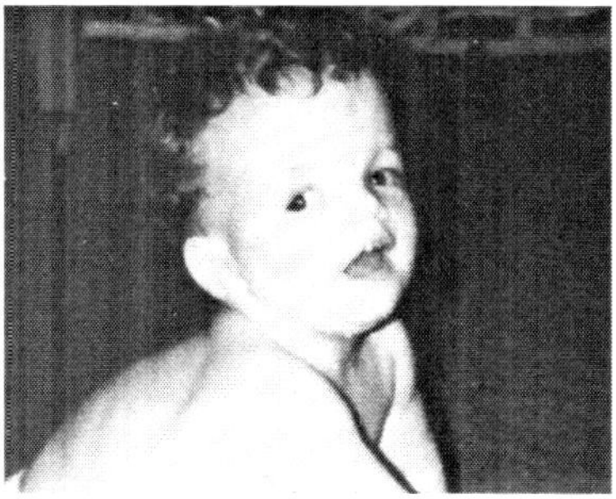

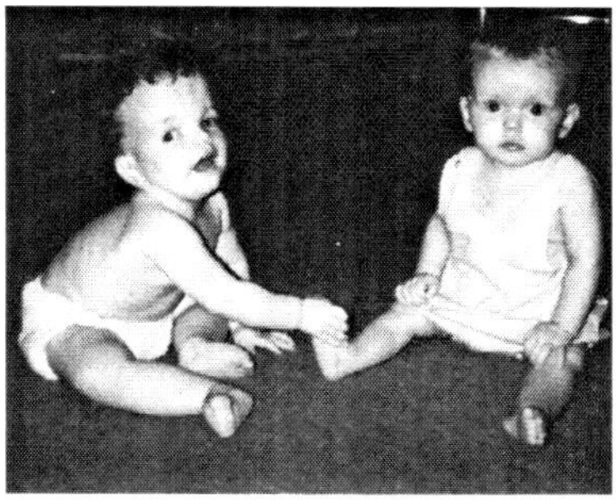

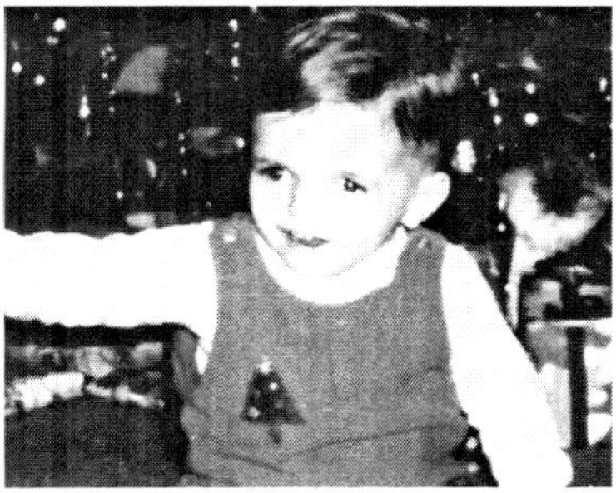

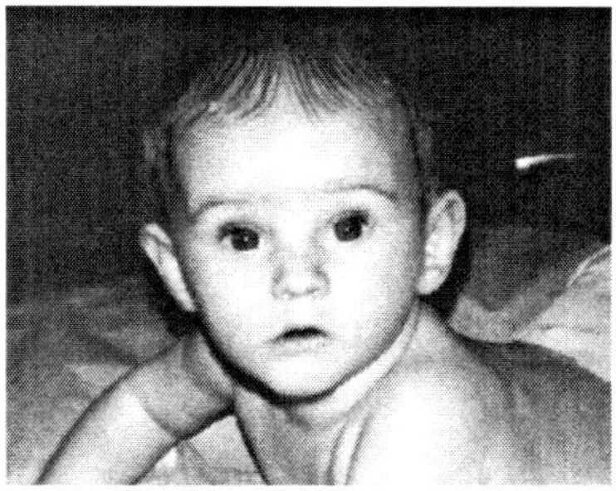

Ann is now a year old and has no semblance of a problem with walking, coordination or intelligence. The lump is better. During the year, I've had pictures taken and have compared Jackie and Ann in different poses. The resemblance is quite remarkable. She does so many things similar to the way Jackie did them. Even likes the same toys.

I think the love and joy and care of this wonderful family as they did the physical things which were necessary was the factor which released Jackie so that he might come back – only with fewer physical problems and with an active mind, but also as a girl so he could laughingly say again, "And Doctor Bel, I luv yu too, In my NEXT life, I'll marry yu!"

CHAPTER FOURTEEN

The New Millennium

The changes which have taken place since the start of this millennium in the field of Obstetrics are truly remarkable.

We've been able to do intrauterine surgery, watch the developing fetus throughout the entire pregnancy, study its responses to stimuli such as sound, touch, and taste, and determine the sex of the baby very early on. I wonder if we've invaded the sacred space of the womb. The Native American people respect all forms of life and never invade another's space without asking permission. They even apologize for cutting a plant or killing an animal for food. They regard each living entity as having an important part in the overall evolving universe and, therefore, it needs its space. We, on the other hand, have such a hunger for knowledge that we have forgotten that with great knowledge comes great responsibility. The responsibility of recognizing and being respectful of boundaries is something that is not even being considered important in our culture. The acquisition of knowledge is vitally important, but not at the expense of ignoring spiritual law. I would suggest that every time we invade the privacy of a developing human being in the womb, we ask permission of not only the mother who we recognize needs to sign a consent form, but also the baby, with great respect, to allow us to view and study the developing process.

This was very early brought to my attention when I had a young woman who wanted to know what the sex of her baby was and the process of ultrasound viewing was just evolving. This was in the early seventies and she had to leave Phoenix and go to Los Angeles in order to have the procedure done. The procedure cost seven hundred dollars which was a great deal of money. She had the money. She felt she needed to know and so she had the procedure done. Much to the amusement of the technician and those around her, this baby at six months absolutely refused to uncross his legs so she could see whether he was a boy or girl. They tried every maneuver they could think of and he refused to uncross his legs so she did not know until he was born that her baby was a boy. As amusing as that story is, it speaks to me of the importance of recognizing the active consciousness of the fetus and that before and throughout the pregnancy it is important for us to create an environment of health and love.

In our scientifically oriented culture, we have developed procedures and technology which is geared towards improving maternal and infant health. Unfortunately, in the process of doing this we have made the birthing process not only a business, but a disease process which requires intervention from the outside much of the time. We have forgotten that women not only have the ability and the knowledge, but they have the power and natural wisdom to deliver babies. This has been known since the beginning of time. We, however, feel that intervention is important and in the process of trying to eliminate some complications have gone way beyond and interfered with the natural process of birthing and have taken the power away from the mother herself and have disrespected the baby's rights. We ignore his or her basic needs.

In 2005 our Center for Disease Control in the United States did a study going back to 1960 of thirty-five different countries regarding infant mortality ratings. In 1960 the United States was listed as eleventh and since that time we have gone down and down until in 2002 we were listed twenty-seventh on this chart with only seven other countries below us in infant mortality ratings. This is truly astounding. We have more technology, more money, more knowledge of the mechanics of birthing than probably any other country and yet we find ourselves getting lower and lower on the list in caring for newborns.

In the year 2005 I was privileged to be part of a team put together by Future Generations to study the maternal mortality in

Afghanistan. At that time it was well known that the maternal mortality rate there was higher than any other place in the world and we really did not know why. My brother, Carl Taylor, M.D., who headed up the Afghanistan division of Future Generations, had been for twenty-five years the head of John Hopkins Department of International Health and then for five years had been the head of UNICEF in China and had been part of the World Health Organization throughout his career. He and his son Daniel Taylor, PhD, started Future Generations which is a nonprofit organization with work being carried on around the world.

We knew that in order to get the information needed we would have to spend time with mature women who had had deliveries. Therefore, after getting permission from their husbands, we set up weeklong workshops where we could spend time living with the women who were the mothers-in-law in the community, and create a pregnancy matrix so that we could track each pregnancy story from each of the thirty-five women who were in the group. This was in the Yakalang town in Bahmian district. These are wonderfully strong women who knew nothing about what happened during a pregnancy. They knew how they got pregnant, but after that it was a mystery. They had taboos about food. They did not give the mother anything to eat or drink after she started in labor until the baby was born and therefore when the time arrived for her to push, she was not only starved, but was hypocalcimic and frequently unable to push the baby out. As a result, they used sever external pressure – anything to get the baby out – resulting in all types of tissue damage, including ruptured uterus, prolapse bladder, severe perineal tears, retained placenta, and hemorrhage.

As difficult as this was to learn, when I came back to the United States and was talking to some of my fellow physicians, I learned that in our country the elective Caesarian section rate, not the necessary, but the elective Caesarian section rate, was thirty-seven percent, much to my horror. What that said to me was that the Afghani women because of their ignorance of the physical aspect of the pregnancy did things that were severely traumatic and detrimental to the mother, and of course, to the baby. But we, who know so much about the body and its physiology, were doing a similar thing except we could sew them up afterwards and the Afghani women were not able to. We were damaging the soul pattern of the mother and the baby. We were taking no thought of the timing which a soul had as to when it was to be born, changing its entire astrological chart and pattern. We, in our ignorance of spiritual law, are causing untold damage to the incoming soul.

The whole situation reminds me of the way conditions were in the late 1940s and early 1950s when Nestle had just come out with formula for the newborn baby. Women were told that the modern woman could do a much better job of feeding their babies if they put them on the bottle with the formula in it. This entailed complicated procedures of sterilizing the bottles and nipples. It required all sorts of different bottles and fancy nipples and special equipment for carrying out these tasks. They were told that in this way the mother knew just how much milk the baby was getting because she could measure it. She knew how many calories and the calculated vitamins and minerals in the formula the baby took in. Nothing was known about the immune system and the hormonal content of breast milk. The babies were thought to be healthier because they were "fat and healthy." The idea that some babies were by nature intended to be lean and strong was considered a myth an "old wives' tale." I wonder how much of the problem we have with obesity in our country may stem from this misunderstood and misused scientific information. The other advantages of breast milk and nursing babies would require another whole chapter in this book. Suffice it to say, we didn't know enough and it was the best of modern science of the time. Women all around the world who were well off and wanted to be the modern woman followed suit and in some places public nursing of babies was banned. I talked myself blue in the face trying to get mothers to nurse their babies during those years, but when a woman wants to be fashionable she has trouble listening to reason.

Try as I may, I cannot come up with any good reason for doing an elective Caesarian section. The Caesarian sections that are necessitated by disproportion or other pathology are different, but to have an elective Caesarian section just for convenience or whatever to me is unconscionable.

Because of the difficult condition we find ourselves in for maternal and infant health regarding pre and perinatal life, the Arizona Health Department has created a task force which has met for the past year to determine what can be done to improve the health of our mothers and babies in Arizona. I am fortunate enough to be part of this task force and we have actively started to help turn this trend around.

Part of our work is reclaiming the sacredness of the womb and acknowledging that pregnancy is not a disease. It is a natural biological process and a family event which is as different and individual as each person born. Birth is a sacred event and the mother and the family need to be supported throughout it. It is now recognized that with the elective C-section there are statistically more deaths or problems with blood clots, more risk of hemorrhage and infection, the possibility of surgical injury, particularly to the bladder, postpartum pain is more pronounced, and the need for narcotics is a hundred percent. On top of all of these complications, the possibility of adhesions forming is much greater. After all, Caesarian section is major abdominal surgery.

There are also risks for the newborn. The newborn is more susceptible to breathing difficulties since there is no activation of the mechanism which naturally occurs during a delivery allowing the baby's lungs to absorb the fluid which is present in the developing lung during the natural process of restriction and release which goes on during a vaginal delivery. Babies delivered by C-section are more apt to have asthma and are more apt to have difficulty with breast feeding.

In this task force we are committed to helping people understand the real risks of the physical complications that are involved with interfering with the natural birthing process (for reasons which are not medically appropriate). Beyond that, there are the unknown complications which can arise from changing the time line which a soul has chosen for herself. We really don't know what we are doing to the astrological pattern, to the evolving growth of that individual soul. I believe that when there is a medical necessity for a Caesarian section, the soul of the mother and of the baby are in tune to why this Caesarian section is being done and adjust to that. But when it is an arbitrary decision, then we are imposing from the outside onto individual souls the time constraint that goes with a birth at that particular moment. The women in Afghanistan did not understand the physical aspects of birthing. We do not understand the emotional and spiritual aspects of birthing and so are causing problems at a level which may be even more profound than the physical complications that go with the birthing process that the Afghani women are using. Pregnancy is not a disease and should not be treated as such. Women have always known how to deliver babies, but we have dis-empowered them. Our lack of confidence in a woman's ability to give birth to a baby is even more humiliating than what we have done to women in the work place or in our search for equal rights. If ever there is a situation in which a woman's rights were taken away, it has been in the arena of obstetrical interference. This has been done through educating with the doctrine of fear, not hope and love. We women have allowed the masculine approach to dominate the way in which babies are born and it is high time that we reclaim our female power and trust the inner knowing which is so much a part of being a woman. As we learn to love ourselves and trust ourselves we will know how and when it is appropriate to acknowledge this power and we will know that each one of us has within us the innate God given wisdom that is part of being a woman. This is our right. It is our privilege and it is our responsibility.

CHAPTER FIFTEEN

In Summary

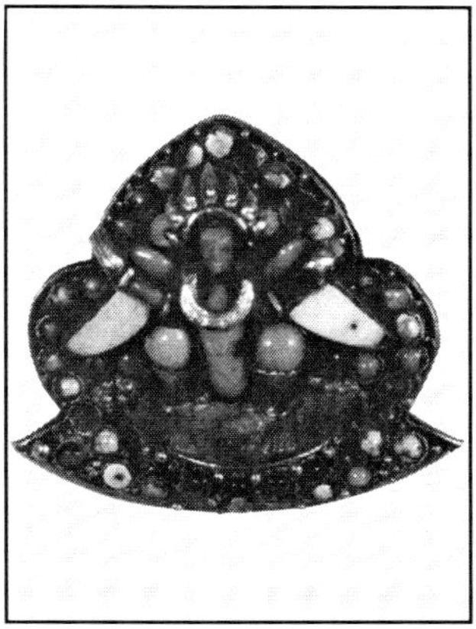

For nearly thirty-five years, I wore a Tibetan pin which my sister gave me when I was matron of honor at her wedding. It was made of brass, rubies, and turquoise, and I always loved this ancient pin, and wore it most of those years without really realizing what it was.

Through the years I went through a series of events with my Tibetan friend which had me puzzled, but which in the end seemed to say something to me about this New Age, and maybe my part in it.

Peter Riddle wore it on the turban he used at our East Indian dinner. This was the first episode. The pin seemingly disappeared. He thought he gave it back to me, but it "reappeared" on his turban a year later, right where he had worn it.

Then we visited an Ashram one day. I was carrying my coat on my arm, and realized that I had lost the pin off my coat. We searched – even with bare feet – all over the property where we had walked. No pin. Maybe we had donated it back to these Eastern Tibetan people. Not so. That evening, before retiring, Bill found the pin in the cuff of his trousers. Had it been there all day?

Next, Bill and I were on our way to San Diego on a plane. The pin was lost again. We searched everywhere around our seat. I checked my purse – it had been on my coat again – and went through my knitting bag piece by piece. No Tibetan pin. We told the airline people about it in case they found it. Bill said, "This time, you've really lost it."

We arrived at the hotel that afternoon, and in the course of unpacking, I looked again in my knitting bag. There, on top of the material I was knitting, on the top of everything in the bag, was my pin.

I looked at that little piece of jewelry that was fashioned in far-off Tibet, and suddenly realized that this was not an ordinary figure. It was a Tibetan woman in labor. Her abdomen was obviously pregnant, her hands were held back, her feet were tied down and she was in a squatting position.

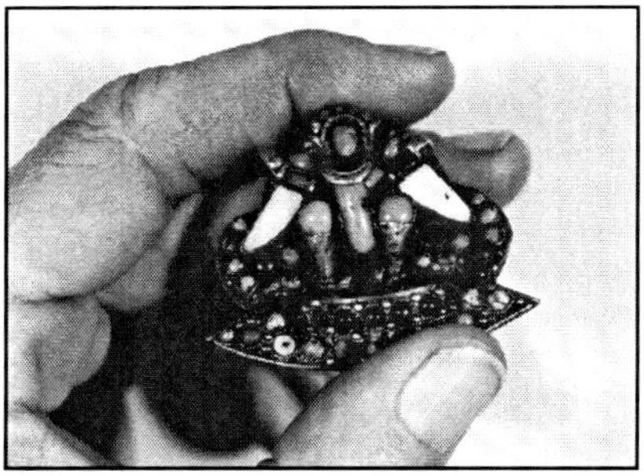

Since that discovery, I've never misplaced or lost that pin. It seemed as if the message had gotten through to me. The message? My life work, no doubt, with the New Age birthing can take a hint from that little Tibetan pin. The New Age may simply be the recovery of memories from times far past, brought up to date and made applicable as consciousness undergoes changes for the better.

There's a new awareness in birthing. Mothers are gaining the privilege of being able to have their babies the way they want to have them. All over the country hospitals have birthing rooms, which allow the mother to remain in one room throughout the process of labor and delivery. Even more than that, she can be in a room she has decorated to her liking, making it as home-like as possible.

Home birthing has come back into vogue, not only here, but in all parts of the nation. Women everywhere are starting to ask why they cannot have their babies at home. Our "Baby Buggy" made such an idea more acceptable to most physicians who were concerned about the dangers that might be inherent with home deliveries.

Nevertheless, home birthing is here once again, and it no doubt is part of the New Age.

There is a new awareness – a new consciousness – in the children being born today. They are a special breed, it seems to me, and they are here with a tough mission to fulfill in today's environment, living in an endangered world.

This generation of souls who are now adults have looked upon war with shame instead of pride. We've had the flower children asking the world to "make love, not war."

Cayce tells in his readings that the entities being born today are only those souls who have sometime in their life experience come to know the "one-ness" of God. These individuals are congregating in the earth again at this time to rekindle the "Christ consciousness" in the world.

There's a new, growing awareness among physicians today, too. More and more doctors are becoming aware of their roles as physicians-priests, and medical organizations are being formed which include this concept clearly in their statements of purpose.

Physicians are recognizing more and more that physical illnesses today, as in ages past, stem from an imbalance in the emotions, an "unrest in the soul," so to speak. Stress plays a major role in the disintegration of the delicate balance between the physical and the mental, creating disease within the body. Stress cannot be avoided, so it must be dealt with. The physician-priest must learn to deal with this problem in a way that goes beyond merely treating the symptom and works with the whole human being, his physical, mental, and spiritual bodies, incorporating the whole person in the process of healing.

In obstetrics and child care, the New Age seems to be saying to us that we must begin to recognize each person as an eternal being, adventuring through one lifetime after another, learning lessons and making contact with others who are learning similar lessons.

Perhaps we may become aware that consciousness is always with us – consciousness of what has happened in the past and what is going to happen. Much as Mr. Cayce said in one reading: "...for all that a soul may experience is visioned as it enters the environ for its experience."

But, let us now allow the thing to happen that Cayce ended that reading with: "Its faith, its hope in individuals as personalities, oft is shattered." (538-30)

The New Age for me is a time of hope, the hope that is such an integral part of the whole healing process, a spiritual quality. And perhaps these stories I've told, the happenings that have become such a vital part of my life and of the lives of others, may provide the kind of hope and love in others' lives that is the earmark of the New Age.

Footnotes

1. Marti-Ibanez, Felix, M.D., "To Be a Doctor," MD, Vol. IV, November 1960, pg. 34.

2. Chamberlain, David, Ph.D., Babies Remember Birth, Jeremy P. Tarcher, Inc., Los Angeles, California, 1988, pg. 103.

3. Ibid, pg. 106.

4. McGarey, William, M.D., Edgar Cayce and the Palma Christi, Edgar Cayce Foundation, Virginia Beach, Virginia, 1970 pg. 111.